# It Gets Easier

# It Gets Easier

**Surviving Twins During
Their First Year**

## TRACEY EGAN

SOUVENIR PRESS

First published in 2016 by Souvenir Press Ltd
43 Great Russell Street, London WC1B 3PD

ISBN 9780285643246

Typeset by M Rules

Printed and bound in Great Britain by Bell & Bain Ltd, Glasgow

# NOTE TO READERS

This publication contains the ideas and opinions of its author. It is intended to provide helpful and informative material on the subjects addressed in the publication. It is sold with the understanding that the author and publisher are not engaged in rendering medical, health or any other kind of personal professional services in the book.

The reader should consult his or her medical, health or other competent professional before adopting any of the suggestions in this book or drawing inferences from it.

The author and publisher specifically disclaim all responsibility for any liability, loss or risk, personal or otherwise, which is incurred as a consequence, directly or indirectly, of the use and application of any of the contents of this book.

# TABLE OF CONTENTS

# ACKNOWLEDGEMENTS

I am deeply grateful to all who supported and encouraged me along the way from the very first idea to the final stages of creating this book, for your belief in me and excitement about my project.

In particular, thanks go to Mr Ernest Hecht and all at Souvenir Press who helped turn my project into a reality. Thanks to my friends for your support and encouragement, and to all who read the manuscript in its earlier versions and accompanying notes. Thanks to my husband, Darren, to my Mum and to Victoria for all your proof-reading and advice. Thanks to Ben and Emily, the inspiration for the book, for being brilliant kids. Thanks to God for giving me such amazing twins, they are absolutely 'wonderfully made' (Psalm 139 v 14)

# INTRODUCTION

Everyone asked if I was shocked when I found out I was having twins. The fact is I *was* completely shocked when I found out. It had simply never ever occurred to me that there could be two babies in there. We turned up for our scan full of anticipation and excitement. We peered at the screen and all I could see was lots of static and the occasional blob and for a wild moment I thought maybe I'm not pregnant at all and the doctor will think I'm crazy. Then I heard my husband asking 'are there two babies?' And indeed there were. Our doctor spent a few moments finding a clearer picture and pointing it all out; there's one and there's the other. I couldn't believe what I was seeing and was glad I was lying down!

Having twins is a mind-blowing experience and nothing in your experience so far will prepare you for your new life plus two. Actually, not much in your friends' experiences with singleton babies will prepare you either because having twins is totally different to having one baby at a time. I know exactly how you feel because I've been there, over the moon and overwhelmed in equal measure. I know what it's like to be awake all day and most of the night, every day and every night. I know what it's like to ask total strangers in the street when things are going to get easier. Like any other new venture in your life this too is a new experience with the steepest learning curve imaginable. It does get easier. It keeps on getting easier. It's also enormous fun and you have two adorable and amazing babies who will bring you more joy than you can ever imagine.

If you feel like you are clueless during those early months with your new twins just remember this; you already know more than you did before the babies were actually born. When the twins are very small it's good to take a moment to remember that and think about all you have achieved. You managed to get yourself dressed today, feed and play with the twins all day, have a cup of tea or coffee, sterilise everything and load up the washing machine. Talk about multi-tasking. When the twins were born you didn't know how you would get them both home from hospital never mind fit in some housework but here you are. And the good news is that it won't always be this hard. In fact, those early months are probably the hardest it will ever be.

When my twins arrived I was given five parenting books, only one of which was about twins and it focused more on the pregnancy than how to survive when the twins arrived. I hope this handbook can be of some use to you during the early months and offers you the reassurance that I know from experience you need: it will all get easier soon.

So, sit down with a mug of tea while you still can and brace yourself for a roller-coaster ride.

# 1

# Congratulations

## CONGRATULATIONS

Firstly; huge congratulations! Has anyone actually said that to you? Or are they too busy telling you how busy you'll be and about their friend's neighbour's cousin who has a two year old and a set of twins and how they can't imagine it . . . If not, then let me say again: huge congratulations. You're having twins! Twins are amazing and will bring you more than 'double the joy'. They are an enormous blessing; fun and so cute and great company for you and for each other. Yes I know they are scary in the beginning. But honestly life gets easier and a whole lot more fun as the months go by.

Having twins is a unique experience. It is fun, busy, and at times overwhelming. My twins brought out in me an entire range of emotions that I wasn't prepared for: profound joy; overwhelming pride; ferocious protectiveness. They scared the living daylights out of me when they were sick. I learned the value of being organised and to ask for, and accept, help. There were some magical moments too, like the first time the twins smiled and gurgled at each other, the first time they smiled and gurgled at me, or the first time they slept through the night.

They are also hard work in the beginning and chances are you will have no idea what day of the week it is or which end is up. When you are in the middle of an Olympic feeding marathon and you've only had two hours sleep you can't imagine that it will ever end. But honestly these crazy early weeks pass and before you know it you'll find yourself saying you wish you could go back to the beginning for a day to see the twins as babies again and just enjoy holding them. Or to be able to nip to the bathroom and know that they will still be in exactly the same spot when you come back! But mostly just to see them that size again and marvel at how cute they were because you really do forget. It can seem never-ending at the time, but I promise it does get easier.

It gets easier and easier by degrees until one day you find yourself relaxing with a cup of tea while the twins are having a nap, and those crazy early weeks and months are a distant memory. I remember asking everyone when it would get easier — good friends, strangers in the street, no-one was safe. I needed to hear that life wouldn't always be this demanding, and that I would get to sleep properly again one day. Life with new twins did gradually get easier and at the same time I got better at dealing with two demanding newborn babies. It gets steadily less difficult as the babies get bigger and stronger and their natural feeding patterns become established and more predictable. So if you take nothing else away from reading these pages, at least remember this one point that I know you need to hear — it will all get easier soon.

## REACTIONS TO THE NEWS

'So were you shocked when you found out you were having twins?' This is usually the first question people asked when I told them. That is, it was the first thing they said after they'd stopped laughing and gasping and clutching either their sides or my arm. 'Wow, twins' they would gasp. 'Are there twins in your family'? It was nearly always the same.

It was fun though and I quite enjoyed having news that surprised people. Because let's face it some or most of your friends and colleagues will have guessed that you are pregnant by the time you break the news officially at twelve weeks or so. Women often guess when their friends are pregnant anyway and this is without having a bigger bump that shows earlier than most. What no-one ever guessed though, was that there were twins on the way. I have to admit I did enjoy telling them and seeing their reactions. There is something great about having a good piece of juicy news to tell your friends, especially when it is happy news like this.

It was also touching how genuinely concerned and helpful people were. Even people I didn't know. My double-sized bump did attract a lot of stares but mostly people were kind and would offer seats and help, and once someone even offered me a lift home as I was walking out of the train station. I know I did look exhausted and huge and I stopped working soon afterwards but it was touching to see genuine concern during rush hour which is usually the craziest time of day.

Your twins will attract attention everywhere you go. Twins are fascinating and few people can resist having a peep, or an outright stare. I grew to enjoy the attention the twins got when we were out and about. It's a little overwhelming at first but it's totally worth going out to the shopping centre for a dose of this goodwill to give you a boost and keep you going. I would beam with pride as other shoppers would declare how cute the twins were and how well they behaved. In queues, lifts, or the chocolate biscuits aisle, the reaction was nearly always the same. First the double take as they try to figure out why the two babies look the same size, then realisation dawns as the look at me and ask 'are they twins?' And I smile and nod and enjoy the attention they are getting.

## WHY TWINS ARE SO GREAT

There are so many reasons to celebrate having twins. Twins have each other to play with. As the months go by, they become more aware and more mobile. They learn to walk together. They learn to talk together. They learn to sit up, crawl, feed themselves and explore their environment together. They discover their favourite cartoons and toys and make up games together. They always have a buddy at the playground, and they always have each other's company at home.

Twins have each other for support. They start looking out for each other from their first day at crèche or mother and toddler group. They will support each other and be there for each other for life and this is a great joy and comfort to us as parents.

Twins are great for lots of practical reasons too. You have two gorgeous babies but only had to endure one pregnancy. Once your babies settle into more predictable patterns you will have one routine, one bedtime ritual, and one set of meals to cook. When your twins are older you will have one drop-off and pick-up at Playschool or Nursery, or school.

## TWIN SCIENCE

Twins can be identical or non-identical. Identical, monozygotic twins develop when one zygote (fertilised egg cell) splits and forms two embryos. They often share the same placenta; they have the same DNA and have different fingerprints and footprints. Non-identical, or fraternal, or dizygotic twins develop when two eggs are each fertilised by two separate sperm cells. They have separate placentas and they are different from each other like any other brothers and sisters.[1]

The birth rate for twins has risen significantly over the last couple of decades for a couple of different reasons. One reason is the rise in availability of fertility treatments and assisted reproductive technology. Medications and hormone treatments can cause more than one egg to be released from the ovaries, leading to fraternal twins. If hormone medications are not successful couples can opt for more complex procedures such as IUI (Intrauterine Insemination) or IVF (In Vitro Fertilisation). During IVF several fertilised embryos are placed directly into the womb, increasing the chance of a successful pregnancy, and also the chances of a pregnancy with multiples.

Another reason for the rise in twin births is that nowadays women tend to wait until they are older to have children. Women over the age of 35 are more likely to produce more than one egg during each cycle, increasing their chance of having fraternal twins[2]. Interestingly, this only applies to fraternal twins; identical twins are rarer and are not affected by the age of the mother.

## TWIN FACTS

There are lots of fun facts about twins. Before long you will have many more to add to this yourself, but in the meantime here are a few for starters ...

- More twins are left-handed than singleton babies[3].
- West African countries have the some of the highest rates of twin births and Hong Kong has one of the lowest[4].
- As many as up to 40% of twins invent their own language[5].

For women, your chance of having twins increases if:

- You are older. Your chance of having twins increases over the age of 35 as your body produces an egg from each ovary[6].
- You have a family history of non-identical twins. If the women in your family have had fraternal or non-identical twins, then there is higher chance that you will too, as there is a tendency to produce that extra egg in your family[7].
- You have had help with fertility medication.
- You are a fraternal twin yourself.
- You eat a certain type of yam. The Yoruba people in West Africa have the highest rate of twin births and they think it may be because they eat a particular type of yam which contains phytoestrogen. It is thought that this phytoestrogen in the yams might boost the ovaries to release two eggs, resulting in more twins[8].

And finally . . . If you already have fraternal twins, you are more likely to have another set of twins next time around, rather than a singleton baby.

## TWIN MYTHS

We all 'know' that twins skip a generation. Or do they? This seems to be a myth because you are more likely to have fraternal twins if your mum had them. This continues from generation to generation and doesn't show any pattern of skipping alternate ones.

Have you heard that twins run in the family? Again however, it seems that it is only non-fraternal ones and not identical ones that can do.

Sometimes people claim that twins are exactly the same. They are not. They are individuals like everyone else with their own individual tastes and likes and dislikes, opinions and personalities and these differences should be nurtured and encouraged.

Twins can also be labelled as the good twin or the bad twin which is incorrect and unfair. Growing up is hard enough without that having labels like that attached.

# Preparing for Twins

## GETTING PREPARED

So how do you prepare for twins? Can you even prepare for twins? It's difficult to picture what it will be like when the twins arrive if you don't have kids and have never experienced looking after two tiny babies at the same time. It is worth giving it some thought though, the more you do in advance, the less panicked and disorganised you'll be when the twins arrive. Everyone keeps telling you how busy you'll be and how little time you'll have, but that's not really all that helpful in terms of helping you to prepare. So here are a few practical things you can do before the babies arrive:

## Action Stations

- Start now before your bump gets too heavy and you get too tired to do too much at a time. Stock your freezer, make lists, rope-in help and gather up all you'll need while you have time and energy.
- Look after yourself well, eat lots and sleep lots.
- There are lots of basic items you can stockpile now like nappies, Vaseline (or similar petroleum jelly), Sudocrem (or similar nappy rash cream), baby wipes and bibs.
- If you are going to use a nappy changing unit why not buy it now and stock it with nappies etc.

- Organise your sterilising equipment and baby bottles and choose your breast-pump if you plan to use one.
- Fill your freezer with meals for after the babies arrive. This is simple to do and you will be so grateful for the ready-made meals later on. Every time you cook, simply double the quantity and pop the extra portions into the freezer.
- Research baby equipment and buy or borrow what you need (see later in this chapter for more about baby equipment).
- Arm yourself with knowledge now while you have time. The more you find out about new babies now, the better prepared you will be for when they arrive and less afraid of your new twins.
- Have fun choosing some baby names.

## Antenatal Classes

Antenatal classes are very helpful for first time mums. Maternity hospitals usually run a programme of classes. The one I attended ran both an all-day course, and a series of five evening courses, as well as refresher courses for second-time-around mums and, most importantly as far as I was concerned, a multiples class. They aim to boost your confidence to help you through pregnancy and child-birth. The more you understand about childbirth and what happens when emergencies arise, the more confident you will be and better able to deal with the whole experience. Hospital-run antenatal classes also have the advantage that they usually include a tour of the labour ward so you can see where you will be going to be spending time later on. Being able to visualise the ward helps you prepare mentally for the birth.

Antenatal classes usually cover all sorts of detail about pain control, signs of labour, and what happens once you go into labour. While these classes are usually geared towards mums expecting single babies, they are still very useful. Don't be put off if your bump is three times the size of everyone else's. The midwife usually waits around at the end of the class to take questions so make the most of this opportunity to find out how everything covered in the class relates to twins.

Multiple Births Associations usually hold antenatal classes specifically designed for parents of multiples. They are run by midwives and often have parents of multiples present to share their experiences too. I strongly recommend attending at least one class and finding out as much as you can now while you have time. It is a fascinating time and once the twins are born you won't have time to read about anything at all for a while, so it's good to read up on it all and arm yourself with knowledge before they arrive.

## Baby Proofing

You can babyproof your home at any time, why not do it before the twins arrive so that you won't have to find the time to do it later on. It is simple to do and shouldn't take you too long.

- Put away anything on the floor, for example stacks of CDs, candleholders and newspapers or books.
- Buy safety catches for your cupboards, especially the one under the sink or wherever you keep your cleaning materials.
- Buy a stair gate for the bottom of your stairs.
- Fit window locks
- Put a fireguard in front of your fireplace.
- Tie down loose cables.
- Buy child safety socket inserts.
- Move your wine rack, or empty it if it cannot be moved.
- Consider putting away or moving anything that you wouldn't want a small child to break such as delicate coffee tables, expensive lamps or ornaments.
- When you are finished sit on the floor and see whether you can reach anything that you wouldn't want your twins to get at, or whether you could bump your head on anything.

## Lower Your Expectations

It is a good idea to lower your expectations about your third trimester. Twin bumps are heavy and twin pregnancy is exhausting. It is very likely that you won't have enough energy to be able to get out and about much during those last few weeks and months. In some cases, mothers expecting twins are prescribed bed rest to relieve pressure on the pelvis or cervix and vital organs, and to conserve energy. You have enough to do and think about without setting unrealistic goals for yourself. I know only too well the feeling of cabin-fever setting in when you haven't been outside in days, never mind fitting in a trip to the hairdressers or anything as exciting as a cafe or a shop. These days are short and will pass in the relative blink of an eye. Aim to only do what you can realistically manage and before you know it you will be past this house-bound stage and back out and about.

## SHOPPING FOR YOU

I'm sure you've realised by now that a twin bump is no ordinary bump. You will probably find that you need to switch to maternity clothes more quickly than your friends did on singleton baby pregnancies. No getting away with wearing old trousers with the top button open for you. In fact, this might be a good time to warn you that your bump will be fairly large by the time the end of your pregnancy rolls around, what with having two babies in there. Chances are you will go through a change or two of maternity clothes, trading up the sizes before the end. I bought a gorgeous pair of maternity jeans at three months pregnant, only to have outgrown them two months later.

Shopping for afterwards is even trickier. By the time the twins came along I was so sick of my maternity gear I was delighted to give it away. There were an awkward couple of months after the twins were born when nothing fit at all. My maternity clothes were too big, and most of my pre-baby clothes were (and still are!) too small. So maybe leave some room in your clothes budget for a trip out to the shops to buy some things to wear after the babies are born. You will get things that fit you properly which will help boost your confidence and the retail therapy will give you a lift.

## SHOPPING FOR THE BABIES

This is the fun part. Who doesn't like shopping for cute little babygros and other teeny tiny baby things? It's hard work too though, when you are pregnant with twins and can't carry very much. Make lists, rope in family to help, and give yourself loads of time. It helps to bear in mind that you will more than likely be given lots of teddies as gifts so, difficult as it to resist the cute stuff, try not to go too mad buying fluffy teddies and concentrate on the things you need.

## Baby Equipment

There is a very wide range of baby equipment available to buy and if you have never had children before it can be quite difficult to figure out how much of it you actually need. There is a bewildering amount of choice out there, some of it essential and some of it frivolous but all of it expensive when bought in one go. Having to buy a crib, cot, nappies, bottles, clothes and a monitor for one baby is pricey enough without having to buy all the same gear for a second baby too. Some of the equipment is only used for a very short time as the twins grow out of things so quickly, so there is a strong case to be made for seeking out good quality second-hand items where possible. Some parents say they spent thousands on kitting out their nursery for twins; others borrowed lots of the gear and got away without breaking the bank. Ultimately it's up to you how much of the equipment you buy and how much you spend on it all. Some things like cribs or Moses baskets are only used for a couple of months so you could consider borrowing them from friends or family. Buying a second hand pram in great condition can also keep the budget down.

Some things are handy to know but you really only figure them out through experience or trial and error. Hopefully I can spare you a bit of time with some little things we figured out the hard way.

### An Extra Kettle

I invested in a second inexpensive kettle so that one could be boiled exclusively for bottles and I never had to worry about anyone else switching the kettle back on to make themselves a cup of tea when I had boiled it up to make a batch of bottles.

### Comfy Seats

Comfy seats upstairs or in the babies' room for doing feeds at night are not essential strictly speaking, but make everything a lot more comfortable in the middle of the night. If you can't actually be in bed then you may as well be in the next most comfortable place you can manage. There's no need to buy a special nursing chair although the new ones in the baby shops can look beautiful. Instead you can either move an armchair into your nursery, or move your baby gear closer to an armchair.

## Cots

There are a few quick tips to keep in mind when choosing your cot.

- Sides that drop down are very handy. It is much easier to change the bedding with the sides lowered and much easier to reach into the cot to sooth your twins if you don't have to stretch too far over the side.
- It is useful to have cots with two mattress heights. When the twins are very small and can't roll around yet you can have the mattress at the higher level so that you don't have to stretch down so far to pick them up. The mattress will be low enough to be a safe height for your twins, but it will be high enough to help to avoid placing too much strain on your lower back. As the babies get bigger you can lower the mattress level.
- Do make sure that the cot rails are close together so that your babies can't stick their heads through them and get stuck.
- Some cots are designed to convert into beds. These cot-beds cost a little bit more initially and are bigger than regular cots but the idea is that they should last for a longer time, usually up to age 4 or 5, and save the hassle of having to buy toddler beds when the babies are ready to move out of their cots and into a bed. Our toddlers were thrilled when the sides were taken off the cots to convert them into beds. The size of the bed is perfect for toddlers and it bought us time to research which kind of 'big bed' we would buy for the next stage.

## Disposable Bottles

You can buy ready-made (disposable) bottles at the hospital for the first week at home if you are bottle-feeding. When you bring your two new hungry babies into the house for the first time, the last thing you want to think about is how to work the steriliser and make up feeds. Handy little ready-made bottles of formula will give you the breathing room you need to get everyone home and settled, and to figure out all of the rest of it in your own time.

## Floor Mats

Many stores sell interlocking foam squares that you can place on the floor to create a softer space for the babies to crawl about in. They are especially useful if you have tiled floors. Some have letters or numbers in each square which look very cute. However, they can be a bit impractical because the twins will just spend their time pulling the letters or numbers out. Plain coloured squares are much more practical.

I do know someone who bought helmets for her twins when they were at the standing up and falling over stage, because she was afraid they would really hurt their heads on the flagstone floors. Mum always knows best and sometimes you really have to improvise. Babies fall a lot during their early toddler stage and foam squares work well to soften up hard surfaces and create a softer landing.

## Medical Supplies

There are a certain number of medical supplies that can be very useful, even essential, for life at home with your new twins. These are some things I couldn't manage without:

- ✓ Thermometer
- ✓ Vaseline or other similar petroleum jelly
- ✓ Sudocrem or other similar nappy rash cream
- ✓ Calpol
- ✓ Baby moisturiser
- ✓ Emulsifying ointment
- ✓ Baby olive oil
- ✓ Baby Wipes
- ✓ Medical wet wipes available from pharmacies for cleaning equipment

*Baby Monitors*

There is a quite a large range of baby monitors out there to suit every budget. The more expensive, the more functions the monitors have.

Basic monitors will usually be digital audio monitors with around a 50m range indoors, and a built-in nightlight. Some might have a couple of channels so you could use a different channel for each baby.

The next level monitors are movement and sound monitors. These have a sensor pad which lies under the mattress and detects even the tiniest movement such as gentle breathing. If no movement has been detected for twenty seconds an alarm will sound. The sensor-pads really are extremely sensitive so if your twins are in their cots the sensor pad will detect them there, even if they are fast asleep. It is designed to give you total peace of mind, for example, on the mornings when the twins sleep in a bit longer, you know they are fine because the sensor-pad can detect their breathing. Just remember to switch the monitor off before you pick up either baby because if you don't the alarm will go off after twenty seconds. These monitors typically come with a built-in nightlight, a longer range and a couple of channels. They also usually have a room temperature display which is surprisingly handy. Babies should not be too warm because they cannot regulate their own temperatures. Room-temperature displays allow you to regulate the temperature in the room.

The top level (i.e. the most expensive) monitors are digital movement and sound monitors which come with a video display so you can see your twins while they sleep. They have a small video screen and an infrared camera so you can see the babies at night. They have room-temperature displays, remote-controlled nightlights, a long range and sensor-pads to go under the mattress which detect movement every twenty seconds. They often have talk-back function too, so that you can talk to your twins from a different room.

We invested in the mid-range Angel-care monitors with sensor-pads under the mattresses. The peace of mind I got from knowing that the babies were fine was worth every penny they cost. I still use them for the room-temperature displays and nightlights even though the twins are no longer in cots. I visited a friend recently who had a video screen with her monitor and we could see her toddler playing in her cot. Very cute, but also very handy, because her toddler then proceeded to have a really long nap and we could see on the monitor that she was fine.

Ultimately it's really up to you which you would prefer and which will suit your budget. All you really need is some sort of device that will let you hear your babies when they cry; the rest is up to you.

*Moses Baskets:*

Moses baskets are ideal for newborn babies to sleep in and have the great advantage that you can easily carry them around from room to room. We carried the Moses baskets downstairs in the morning so that the twins could nap downstairs during the day. We would carry them back upstairs again in the evening for night-time. It turned out that this also had the unexpected and really useful side effect of creating a separation between day and night which eventually helped the twins to distinguish the difference between the two.

You can buy fitted sheets that fit the Moses baskets although these are not essential as folded cot sheets will do the job just as well. You can also buy stands for the baskets to sit on which allows you to reach the babies more easily and avoid placing strain on your lower back.

*Nappy Bin*

A separate dedicated nappy bin is a great idea. Twins generate a lot of soiled nappies between them so it can be very useful to have a separate nappy bin for them all. The bins are specifically designed to wrap each nappy in plastic wrap so you don't have to suffer the nappy smells. The bin liner comes in a specifically designed cartridge and you can buy replacements in many stores.

*Prams*

There is a vast selection of prams on the market. Fortunately there is less choice for twins making the selection process a little easier.

There are double buggies with seats side-by-side, or tandem buggies with seats front and back. The double buggies have improved a lot over the years and are not as wide as they used to be. Some have three wheels, are very easy to manoeuvre and are suitable from birth. Tandem prams have seats one in front of the other. They are narrower than their side-by-side cousins although they are longer and can be slightly heavier depending on the model. Some are suitable from birth and adaptable for use throughout the various stages from tiny newborns to bouncing toddlers.

It can be very difficult to decide which type of pram to go for. There are a few simple questions to consider which can help narrow your selection and ultimately choose the right 'travel system' for you.

- How wide is your front door? Websites and brochures usually display measurements for their prams and buggies. Some side-by-side buggies can be quite wide, if it doesn't fit comfortably through your front door and takes up your entire hallway, then maybe it's not the one for you.
- Will the pram fit into your car boot? Ask for the measurements of the pram or buggy folded down and check that it will fit into your car boot.
- Will you spend much time in your car? If yes, then a pram which holds the car seats would be ideal. Some travel systems have adapters that enable you to interchange car seats and buggy seats. You can lift the twins straight out of the car still snug and snoring in their car seats and then click these onto the pram frame. No need to disturb anyone if you want them to stay asleep. It is also faster to lift the car seats out of the car and click them onto the pram frame than it is to take the twins out of their car seats and strap them into the pram.
- Will you spend more time walking than driving? If you will spend much more time on foot and only driving occasionally then a lighter side-by-side stroller with three wheels for extra manoeuvrability might be the one for you. There's no need to spend money on a pram which takes the car seats if you will be walking most of the time.
- How long will you be using this pram for? Some pram

systems include larger buggy seats for when the twins get a little bigger and can sit up by themselves. Once they have outgrown the little carry cot or tiny baby seats you will need to either change over to the bigger buggy seats or buy a different stroller.

- Would you prefer new or second-hand? If you don't mind buying second-hand you can get some great bargains. A lot of people sell on their prams once they have finished with them. If you do buy second-hand, make sure you see the pram first and check that all parts are included and in good working order. Check the pram wheels and brakes are still working well.

## Sterilisers

Sterilising your twins' feeding equipment is also mentioned in Chapter 5 but I wanted to include it here so that you had a list of all your baby equipment in one place.

Most steam sterilisers fit up to six bottles. Basic ones fit into most microwaves and take several minutes to sterilise six bottles (times vary depending on the steriliser and microwave wattage). These bottles remain sterilised for up to three hours as long as the lid is unopened. Take care when opening the lid as the steam can be very hot.

Electric sterilisers are slightly more expensive. Bottles remain sterilised for up to six hours as long as the lid remains unopened.

Digital sterilisers also steam the bottles, but have the advantage that you can remove a single bottle and press a button to re-sterilise the remaining bottles. No need to remove everything and start all over again, and you have five more bottles ready for when you need them.

Other sterilising methods include boiling the bottles and teats in a pan for ten minutes, or placing the bottles and equipment in cold water which has a sterilising solution dissolved in it.

Whichever method you choose, make sure to wash all bottles and equipment thoroughly before sterilising and follow the manufacturer's instructions carefully.

*Travel Booster Seats*

Travel booster seats are very handy to have in the boot of the car if you are visiting friends or relatives during the day. Most people don't have spare high chairs lying around so it can be useful to have small travel ones to bring with you. These seats can be attached to dining room chairs and hey-presto, you have two high chairs for your twins to sit in and join in with everyone for lunch. They are by no means essential though, so ideally borrow some if you need them, or find some second-hand ones in good condition.

*Travel Cots*

Travel cots are also very handy to have if you think you will stay away overnight with your twins. It is a good idea to check out the cot measurements before you buy anything as some travel cots can be quite small. There are some larger ones that will last you for longer, but you might want to check that they will fit into the boot of your car before you purchase one.

One of the biggest problems with travel cots is that two of them can take up storage space in your house so maybe only invest in them if you think you will be doing a lot of travelling. Most hotels have travel cots nowadays so you really only need them for visiting relatives when the twins are small.

## BEING PREGNANT WITH TWINS

Twin pregnancies follow the same patterns as singleton ones. The key difference is the obvious one, there are two babies growing instead of one. You may have some of the same pregnancy symptoms as with a singleton pregnancy such as tiredness, nausea and vomiting, although these can be more severe when you are expecting twins.

So how do you cope if you have any of those symptoms and are working full-time? The truth is that it can be difficult. I was extremely tired throughout the pregnancy, all my resources were going into growing two babies and I had very little energy leftover.

Working was a huge struggle and I used to have a nap when I got home in the evening before dinner because I was just so tired. I took to buying a hot chocolate on the way to work every morning (it was winter-time) to take my mind off the journey and got the occasional taxi from the train station to the office. You'll find your own way to cope with it but here are a few things to remember in the meantime:

- When you are busy at work it can be easy to let hunger and tiredness creep up on you. Try to keep a supply of healthy snacks to hand to keep you going in-between meals.
- Try not to plan too much for your evenings. You'll be too tired to do anything anyway and need to rest as much as you can.
- Talk to your doctor and your HR officer to see whether working part-time might be an option for you for the last month or two.
- You can always start your maternity leave early if you have to. If you are just too tired it might be the sensible thing to plan to stop a bit earlier and give yourself the rest you need. Your body is working incredibly hard growing your twins, why place extra strain on it if you don't have to.

## Baby Development through the Trimesters

### The First Trimester

During these weeks the embryos develop and form into tiny babies. By week twelve all the vital organs are developed and they usually have formed fingers, toes, eyelids and even finger nails. All the bones have formed although they are still soft and your twins can move around although you won't be able to feel this yet.

While you may know you are pregnant, you may not be aware at this stage that you are expecting twins. Most people don't find out about the second baby until they have their first scan at around twelve weeks.

### The Second Trimester

During this trimester the babies' vital organs and digestive and nervous systems develop and mature. Most people have a long scan at around twenty weeks or so. During this scan your twins are examined in great detail to check that they are developing normally.

By twenty-four weeks the babies are very active and may even have hiccoughs as their chests and lungs make breathing-like movements. They can now hear you and teeth have started to grow. By twenty eight weeks the babies can open their eyes. They are developing muscles and putting on weight all the time. By the very end of the second trimester your twins will start to have a higher chance of survival if born prematurely.

Your bump will also be much larger than friends who are having singleton babies and you may start to notice stretch marks. Your legs might start cramping and some people say they feel warmer than they normally would. Iron levels usually take a dip around this stage too so your doctor will recommend you take an iron supplement. Don't be afraid to try a few until you find one that suits you. I tried four different preparations before I settled on one that didn't affect me too badly. This one had vitamin C in it which helps the body absorb the iron. If you don't like the first one you try, don't suffer in silence, move on and try another one.

### The Third Trimester

By the start of third trimester the twins are growing hair and their eyelids are starting to open. Their brains are developing rapidly and eyebrows and eyelashes might be visible. At thirty-two weeks both babies can see and hear and react to loud noises. By thirty-six weeks the twins' lungs are developing faster than those of singleton babies as they tend to be born earlier. They are developing reflexes and are growing hair. Twin pregnancy is considered to be full-term at thirty-eight weeks.

During this last trimester the babies grow big and heavy and you will feel a lot of pressure in your pelvis from the weight of the babies. Expect to feel very tired and don't be surprised by haemorrhoids, ligament pain, heartburn, and a bladder that needs to be emptied very frequently. As the babies grow even bigger you may experience shortness of breath and back pain, and difficulty finding a comfortable position can make it hard to sit or sleep. Make sure your hospital bag is packed as you could go into labour at any time.

It is normal to have more check-ups and scans during this trimester than your friends with singleton pregnancies. Twins are usually monitored closely to make sure they are growing and developing as they should.

## WHAT TO BRING TO HOSPITAL

For first time mums it is very hard to know what to bring to hospital. You haven't done this before so how do you know what to pack? The answer is: keep it simple. If you find out when you get there that you need something from home your partner or family can fetch it for you, or bring it with them on their way in the next day. The general advice is to pack three bags, one for the labour ward if you are having the twins naturally, one for your stay in hospital, and one for the babies. Most labour wards are limited for space so patients would normally be advised to just bring a few essentials in the labour bag and get someone to bring everything else in a suitcase afterwards. Don't forget your baby car-seats as you won't be able to come home without these.

### The Labour Bag

- ✓ 1 × nightdress (most people I know bought a huge cheap one that they could chuck away afterwards)
- ✓ 1 × clean nightdress for afterwards
- ✓ Slippers or flip-flops — something very comfortable as your feet can swell at this time
- ✓ Bottle of water
- ✓ Socks — you could be hanging around for a while and a lot of people find their feet can get cold
- ✓ A few toiletries such as moisturiser, toothbrush and toothpaste, and something to tie back your hair
- ✓ Change for the parking meter

## Hospital Bag

- ✓ Clean nightdresses or pyjamas
- ✓ Light dressing gown (it is usually very warm on the wards)
- ✓ Slippers
- ✓ Wash bag and toiletries
- ✓ Maternity sanitary towels
- ✓ Breast pads (for leaks even if you are bottle feeding)
- ✓ Baggy clothes for going home

## Babies Bag

- ✓ 10 babygros per baby
- ✓ 10 vests per baby
- ✓ Nappies
- ✓ Baby wipes
- ✓ Vaseline and Sudocrem
- ✓ Lots of bibs or muslin cloths whichever you prefer. But you can never have too many
- ✓ Blankets for going home
- ✓ Baby hats for going home

## THINGS THEY DON'T TELL YOU

Being pregnant is a unique experience and nothing prepares you for it. There are many things you only find out when you are pregnant and you wonder how you didn't know this before. There are more things you only find out after the babies arrive that you didn't know either. I call these 'the Things They Don't Tell You'. I include these so that you can feel slightly more prepared and above all you can rest assured that you are not the only one that didn't know something that has suddenly become obvious. Or maybe I was just very naive and these things are blindingly obvious to everyone else. In any case here are a few things you probably already know —

1. You will need to buy bigger underwear a few times as you stretch and grow.
2. Pregnancy rashes are common.

3. Your bones can relax and stretch a bit — and this also affects your feet. I couldn't wear some of my favourite heels after the twins were born because they simply didn't fit anymore. However it did provide me with the ultimate excuse to go and buy new ones.

4. Some risks such as premature birth, gestational diabetes and pre-eclampsia are higher in multiple pregnancies. Watch out for anything unusual and have regular prenatal check-ups. Speak to your doctor or prenatal health care team if you have any concerns.

5. Some people say it took them a little while to bond with their babies. In the movies the heroine bonds with her babies immediately, in real life it can take a little bit longer. If you feel a bit surreal on that first day don't worry because you are not the only person who has ever felt like that. If it continues after a couple of days though you should talk to someone about it.

6. You will cry after the babies are born. Maybe not straight away, or even for a few days, but definitely at some point around day three or four. The tears may dry up after a few days or may last for a few weeks. This is just hormones and totally normal.

7. Even if you choose to bottle feed your poor sore boobs will still leak. Again, I know this shouldn't be a surprise, but it was.

8. You will have conversations about wee and poo. Yes, you will. Not only that, but you won't believe how much you will find to say on the subjects. I used to be a bit shy about discussing matters relating to toilet functions. So it is with great amusement that I have found myself having fairly in-depth discussions about my babies' nappies. The frequency, size, shape, colour, quantity, consistency, and smell of the nappies' contents are all topics for discussion — nothing is sacred.

9. Your perspective will change. You will see the world in a new light and all of the things your parents used to say to you will suddenly make sense. In fact, you may even actually turn into your parents.

10. You will start to forget things. Your overworked brain can't hold *that* much information. Make notepads and pens your new best friends.

*And finally . . . If you think you are alone don't worry, it's the same in every house. I know it can look like some people have things completely under control and never have a moment's trouble or stress, but they were new to all of this and had to learn how to cope with it in the same way that you are doing. Even though we are all individuals, we still go through similar things at this stage and the emotions, the stress, the sleep deprivation and the hectic schedules are completely normal and more common than you think.*

# Brace Yourself: The Twins are Coming!

## WHEN TO GO TO HOSPITAL

How do you know when it is time to go into hospital? Do you race into the hospital at the first sign of a twinge around your due date, or do you wait until you are out of your mind with painful contractions to go? Every mother will have a different story about their experience (and revel in the telling of it) and you can bet each story will be different. So how do you know when it's the right time for *you* to go?

Many labours start with labour pains or contractions. Once the pains last for around 40 seconds each and are ten minutes apart or less you should go to the hospital. Mind you, if you live a distance away you might want to set off earlier.

You might have a 'show' although not everyone has this. A 'show' is a plug of mucus with a tiny amount of blood staining. It can often be accompanied by lower back pain or abdominal discomfort. This lets you know that labour will be starting soon but you are not in labour yet.

Alternatively the first sign of anything happening might be when your waters break. Once your waters break you should go into the hospital even if your contractions have not started.

It can be difficult to decide when to set off for the hospital. You are the best person to know what is going on with your body at that moment and you can always phone up and talk to the hospital staff about it if you aren't sure. The main rule is, if you are in any doubt at all, or suspect you might have a problem, you should go to the hospital straight away. Problems might be things such as:

- Bleeding
- Severe headaches or visual disturbances
- Your baby is not moving as much as usual
- Your fingers and feet become very swollen

Remember, it is better to be cautious and go to hospital too early, than to wait at home until it is too late.

## PAIN RELIEF

There are several different types of pain relief available and the staff in the hospital will discuss your options with you. There are no prizes for suffering in silence so if you are in pain speak out.

### Entonox (Gas and Air)

Entonox is half oxygen and half nitrous oxide and has a calming effect. It can help numb the pain a little bit but doesn't block it completely. The gas is inhaled through a mouthpiece and takes 30 seconds to build up enough gas in your system before you feel any relief. Start to breathe in the gas as soon as you feel a contraction start.

Entonox has the advantages of being relatively quick and easy to use, and you can use it by yourself having to wait for help. It leaves your system as soon as you stop taking it so it has no lasting effects and is safe for your twins.

Entonox can also have unpleasant side effects. Some people say it makes them feel nauseous and woozy and dries their mouth out. It can take a while to get the hang of it too so it might take a while before you get any benefit from it. It doesn't take the pain away but might help you relax and cope with the pain better.

### Pethidine

Pethidine is a morphine based painkilling drug. It helps you to relax and the more relaxed you are the better you will deal with the experience. It is usually given in the form of an injection and the affects last for a couple of hours. The biggest disadvantage of

Pethidine is that it crosses into the placenta and can make the babies sleepy. Other disadvantages include dizziness and vomiting in some cases.

## TENS

TENS machines are used during the early stages of labour. They are small devices and have wires with electrodes on the ends which you attach to your back. They are designed to emit small currents which block the pain by prompting your body to produce endorphins. You control the pulses and how long you use it for. It has no known side effects either for you or your babies but might take a little while to build up. Some people love these little machines, others think they don't work very well. If you don't think yours is doing anything for you just take it off.

## Epidural

An epidural blocks pain in your lower body while you stay fully conscious. It works by preventing the pain signals from travelling from your uterus along your spine to your brain. It blocks out pain but doesn't totally block out sensation, so if you have a Caesarean Section you can still feel some pulling and pushing without feeling any pain.

The epidural is given by the anaesthetist. You will be asked to lie still on your side while they insert a local anaesthetic and the epidural tube into your spine in your lower back. You will be able to sit up again after this is finished. You and the babies will be monitored very closely.

Epidurals give very effective pain relief in labour and have the advantage that you are still awake the entire time. It is likely to make your legs feel heavy or numb though so you will have to stay in bed.

## Spinal Block

Sometimes twins can both lie in a breach position and in this case you would be scheduled for an elective caesarean. Spinal blocks are usually given for these procedures and take effect faster than epidurals. They can be effective in five minutes and last for around two hours. It also differs from an epidural in that it is injected directly into the spinal fluid, instead of into the space around the spinal cord.

It has all of the advantages of an epidural in that you will be alert during the operation and awake to meet your babies when they are born. It provides total pain relief although you will still be able to feel some movement.

## LABOUR

### Natural Birth

I know you're probably nervous about labour — you wouldn't be human if you weren't — but a natural birth is the option with most advantages. The main one being that you won't have had major surgery and will be up and about on your feet relatively quickly again. You will be able to pick up the babies straight away and will be able to drive as soon as you feel like it.

Having twins by natural delivery does not mean having to go through the entire labour twice. You will have to deliver babies twice at stage two, but will only go through stage one once. In fact, the early stages are very similar to 'singleton' labour, with the exception that you will have a second baby to deliver after the first. The good news is that many women report that the second twin is actually easier to deliver than the first one because the cervix is fully dilated by then and the first baby has already done the hard work. You will be monitored very closely throughout the whole procedure. It is also usually recommended that you give birth to your twins in hospital because of the risks involved. In addition, it is quite common for one of the twins to spend a little bit of time in special care.

### Stage 1

Stage 1 is usually the longest stage. However, most people delivering twins by a natural birth will only experience this stage once, similar to women having one baby.

Stage one starts with contractions lasting up to forty-five seconds that can be up to an hour apart. In fact, you may not even be aware of them in the beginning. When the contractions are ten minutes apart go to your hospital where you will be admitted to the labour ward. Contractions continue to speed up until they last more than a minute and come as often as every second minute. You might start to feel an urge to push, but you must resist this until your doctor or midwife tells you to do so.

### Stage 2

By stage two your cervix is fully open and the first baby enters the birth canal. Your doctor or midwife will guide you, telling you when to push and helping the baby out. Once the first baby has been born there is usually a short pause for up to about fifteen minutes. If the second twin is in a good head-down position you will be guided through the pushing process again. In most cases this is easier the second time around as your cervix is already fully open and your birth canal has already been stretched.

### Stage 3

During stage three the placenta is delivered. This usually involves a few smaller pushes although the medical team usually assist the process to speed things up and prevent you losing too much blood.

### Apgar Score

The medical team will assess each baby's 'Apgar Score'. This is a test performed on all newborn babies to assess their colour, heart rate, muscles, reflexes and breathing. The second twin will often have a lower Apgar score than the first twin, but this is quite normal.

## CAESAREAN SECTION

A caesarean section is the birth of the baby by surgery. You might be planning or hoping to have the twins naturally but do be prepared for the fact that caesarean sections are necessary in certain circumstances. They can be planned beforehand or performed because of an emergency during labour. The main reasons why a caesarean might be necessary are:

- If the babies are lying horizontally
- The baby's feet, bum, or shoulders enter the birth canal first
- The umbilical cord comes through your cervix
- The babies show any signs of distress
- Labour is too slow or stops

Try not to worry though. If a caesarean section is necessary for you, it is because it is the best and safest option for both you and your twins.

## ELECTIVE CAESAREAN

Although natural delivery is considered the best option for recovery, it is not always possible for everyone to have one. If your babies are lying in a breech position or your placenta is positioned across the neck of your womb you will be scheduled for an elective caesarean. You would also be scheduled for this surgery if you had pre-eclampsia, high blood pressure, diabetes, or some other medical condition, or if you have had a caesarean section before.

You and your partner or whoever you have supporting you will be brought into theatre separately. You will be brought in first and given your spinal block (like an epidural only faster). You will be given a small drink of an antacid solution to neutralise the acid in your tummy. You will be hooked up to a drip for fluids and medication and will have a catheter inserted. A screen is erected over your tummy so you can't see what is going on although you are fully awake so you can hear everything, quite a surreal experience. Your partner is brought in last and sits beside your head so they can't see anything either.

There will be a lot of people in the room while the operation takes place. Besides you, your partner, and your consultant or surgeon, there will be nurses, midwives, paediatricians, assistant surgeons, an anaesthetist and maybe some other trainee doctors.

You do hear everything during the surgery as you are fully conscious. This is a little disconcerting if you are not prepared for it — surgery is a noisy affair and you can hear it all even though you don't feel any pain. You hear clinking instruments, monitors beeping, suction, muffled voices and then through it all the first twin's first cry. You can also hear all the activity in the background as the first twin is weighed etc while the second one is being born. It's a bizarre and overwhelming experience to be operated on at the same time as you are meeting your twins for the first time.

When they are born the consultant will hold them up for you to catch a quick glimpse before the paediatrician takes them to one side to check that everything is okay. Meanwhile the second twin is born and checked to make sure they are okay too. Assuming everything is fine they are wrapped up and brought to you and your partner for a few moments.

You will be brought up to a recovery room for a while after the operation and then moved down to a ward to reunite with your babies and partner later on.

You might think that a caesarean section would be preferable or easier than enduring a natural birth with twins. There are some downsides though. A caesarean section is a major operation and has all of the disadvantages of any normal surgery. You stay longer in hospital and have the usual risks of post-op infection, bleeding, and blood clots. You will experience some pain and it will take you at least 4—6 weeks to recover from the operation. Your core strength takes a beating — in fact it will be non-existent afterwards and as a result you may experience back pain.

I don't mention this to worry you, or cause any panic. If your consultant recommends a caesarean section for you, then it will be because it is the safest way to deliver your babies. I only mention the downsides to the surgery to give you the fullest picture of what happens in case you are thinking of requesting an elective caesarean.

## TIPS TO HELP RECOVER AFTER CAESAREAN SECTION

It will take up to six weeks to recover from the surgery. Recovery is difficult because you don't have time to rest and pamper yourself in the same way you would have done before having two newborn babies demanding your attention. No lying around on the sofa under a duvet drinking hot chocolate and watching back episodes of your favourite television programmes for you!

You will experience some discomfort at first and should take care of yourself to help speed recovery and prevent infection. You are actively discouraged from lifting immediately after surgery and to try to keep lifting to a minimum for up to six weeks afterwards. Needless to say, this can make life quite awkward for you when you have new twins to look after. It is very tempting to do too much yourself, whether through a desire to be independent or frustration at having to let others do most things for you. Remember, if you do too much, you risk slowing down the healing process and causing infection to the wound.

It is so important to try and follow all of the common-sense guidelines initially to give yourself the best chance of recovery. There are lots of steps you can take to help you through these early weeks.

–   **Accept all the help you can get from nurses in the hospital.**
    They will teach you how to hold, feed, change, and bathe your babies. They may even mind them at night for you so you can get some precious and much needed sleep.

–   **Take it as easy as you can.**
    I know this is funny when you consider how busy having twins can be. Let visitors put the kettle on for themselves. They won't mind and will be more than happy to make tea for you and feel helpful at the same time. You need to take it easy to let yourself heal and avoid infecting the wound.

- **Get help at your house.**
  You will need help with cleaning because besides not having any time to do it, you will be physically weaker than before and won't be able to lift and carry a heavy vacuum cleaner about the house.

- **Be organised.**
  The best way to do this is to think things through. For example, if you live in a two-storey house keep nappies, wipes, creams, blankets, baby clothes et cetera downstairs as well as upstairs to avoid too many trips up and down the stairs. Similarly, consider having Moses Baskets downstairs so that you can live downstairs all day and avoid carrying babies upstairs for naps. Set everything up before you go to hospital to save time when you get home.

- **Fill the freezer with meals**
  It is so important to have hot meals, not only for your physical recovery, but a hot meal will boost your morale after a long hard day and give you strength to face the next one.

- **Do your research**
  If you are breastfeeding it is a good idea to do as much research as possible and talk to friends to find out all their tips. Specialised u-shaped pillows are designed to take the pressure off your abdomen. Similarly breastfeeding lying down achieves the same thing and you get to put your feet up at the same time.

- **See a physiotherapist before you leave the hospital**
  They will show you some gentle exercises that you can do immediately after you get home which will help strengthen your abdominal muscles and help maintain circulation. Ask about abdominal support bandages to give your lower back some extra support.

- **Drink peppermint tea**
  During the days after your surgery your digestive system
  might feel sluggish and you may experience painful trapped
  wind. Peppermint tea is very effective in relieving
  discomfort. Ask your nurse for some, and if it isn't
  available ask your partner or family to pop into the local
  supermarket for some for you.

- **Good lifting technique**
  Your legs should take the strain and not your back. Keep
  your feet shoulder-width apart, bend your knees, and hold
  whatever you are lifting close to you. If you feel a strain in
  your back stop and get someone else to lift it for you.

- **Walk around**
  I think I took too long to get up and moving about. It does
  really lift your spirits to get up and move about even if it's
  just a few steps down the corridor. It also helps get rid of
  painful trapped wind. In fact, the Mayo Clinic say that
  walking around helps the healing process[9].

- **Arrange lifts**
  You will be unable to drive until after your six-week check
  up. If this is going to be a problem for you try to arrange lifts
  before you go into hospital so that you have one less thing
  to worry about when you come home.

- **Accept that you can't do it all**
  Acceptance of your own physical limitations is a key part
  in helping you relax and recover and adapt to your new
  situation. If you expect too much from yourself you will
  only set yourself up to fail and make yourself feel low,
  instead of feeling good about all you have accomplished,
  like learning how to look after two newborn babies at
  once.

- **Don't let it get you down**
  You will recover soon and it will all get so much easier.

– **Wound Care**

The hospital staff will no doubt advise you on how to care for your wound during the first six weeks (or until it has healed). The golden rules were drilled into me by my nurses and are really just common sense but here they are:

---

**DO**

- *Keep your wound clean;*
- *Have a shower or bath every day. Use unperfumed soap or shower gel, taking care not to apply it directly to the wound itself*
- *Dry your wound straightaway and try to keep it as dry as you can*

**DON'T**

- *Touch the wound unless you really have to.*
- *Change your dressings unless told to do so by your doctor or nurse.*
- *Apply any creams or any other products to the wound unless specifically advised to do so by your doctor.*
- *Visit swimming pools, saunas, Jacuzzis etc.*

---

Your nurses and midwives will also talk you through how to tell if the wound is infected. The main signs to watch out for are:

- You have a fever
- The wound is more swollen or sore than usual
- The wound is oozing any type of fluid
- The wound starts to smell unpleasant or bad
- The skin around the wound is becoming red

# The Crazy Early Weeks

## FIRST DAY AT HOME

It is true that there is nothing in life that prepares you for that moment when you arrive home from hospital with your new twins. After the safety and warmth of the hospital you are suddenly all on your own with no trained nursing staff around. It's terrifying, daunting, and overwhelming, and you feel an enormous weight of responsibility. The babies are just days old, you are recovering physically, your hormones are all over the place, and you have to figure out how to use all this new baby equipment and all away from the protection and safety of the maternity ward.

I remember the moment well; it's hard to forget. I could barely walk after the caesarean section a few days earlier, the weeps had set in, I had no clothes that fit although that was the least of my concerns, the babies were due a feed and I hadn't figured out how to work the sterilisers or how to make bottles. It's funny now looking back at it, and I'm sure that if I had to go through it all again I'd handle it all very differently. I like to think I'd be cool and calm and more organised and not so terrified. But as a first time mum recovering from surgery and still in shock at suddenly having two babies I couldn't say I was any of those things.

The good news is — it doesn't get any harder, it only gets easier. It gets easier as you get stronger and your body heals and your hormones return to normal. It gets easier as you learn how to use all of the equipment and grow more confident at changing nappies and feeding and winding the babies. It also gets easier week by week as the babies grow and start to settle down into more predictable feeding and sleeping patterns. I used to ask everyone to tell me that it would get easier! It does, honestly.

## VISITING HOURS

I'm not too sure why I thought I could handle having all of my in-laws to visit on my first day home from hospital with twins five days after major surgery. I was overwhelmed by the twins, the recovery from surgery and the physical exhaustion that comes with that, not to mention not having had much sleep in the last few days, and a body full of alien hormones. At the same time I wanted to show off our amazing babies and I knew the family wished us well and wanted to see the twins. They were all going to want to see the babies sooner or later so I suppose it got that first introduction out of the way.

On the other hand, I know people who have had one baby and who have asked friends and relatives to delay their visits for a little while until everyone finds their feet. With twins it certainly took me a while to find my feet. You can judge for yourself how to manage your visits but there is no shame in spacing them out. There is a lot to be said though for having company and the extra pair of hands is always a help. The company of visitors will help keep your feet on the ground and boost your well-being. Maybe in smaller doses though, and not all at once! Ultimately, it's your say, do what's best for you and your family.

## NAPPIES

### Changing Nappies

Changing nappies quickly becomes an easy and relatively quick if somewhat tedious chore. I only say 'tedious' because with twins you have so many nappies a day to change. It can also be fun and a chance to chat and make funny faces and noises and another job done to tick off the list. Changing nappies in the beginning on the other hand, is a multi-tasking feat of skill followed by a feeling of great accomplishment. There are nappies, cotton wool balls, wipes, Vaseline, and nappy rash creams to juggle. Babies have a habit of letting their heels fall into the nappy so to avoid smearing the nappy contents everywhere it's a good idea to hold onto the ankles with one hand while you juggle everything else with the other. They also have a habit of peeing the second the old nappy comes off so have wipes or a hand-towel or something ready just in case.

Some babies don't like having their nappy changed. They don't like the exposure and feel insecure. If you chat and sing to them the sound of your voice will both distract them and help them feel more secure and make the whole experience more fun. Try and catch their eye as much as possible to reassure them. This takes practice when you are also trying to watch what you are doing, keep their heels out of the nappy, look for wipes and Vaseline, and look at the other twin occasionally to include them and see what they are up to. See why I said you would be multi-tasking?

You will spend quite a lot of time changing nappies with twins so it's a good idea to make things as easy for yourself as possible. To simplify it all here's a list of handy things to have ready and a few tips to help along the way:

- A dedicated changing station is very useful as you can have all of your changing paraphernalia in one place. They also tend to be hip/waist high depending on how tall you are so you can stand up to change the nappies and don't place as much strain on your back. Just make sure your babies can't roll off the stand and never leave them unattended.
- Check that you have everything you need before you start so that you don't have to go hunting for spare wipes or Vaseline mid-way through a nappy change.
- If the phone rings or the doorbell goes either ignore it or bring the baby with you, preferably with a towel wrapped around them as they are likely to pee all over you if you haven't got their nappy on in time.
- Twins generate a lot of dirty/wet nappies between them so I found it very useful to have a dedicated nappy bin. They are designed to contain both the nappies and their smell and I highly recommend getting one. The bin liner comes in a

specifically designed cartridge and you can buy replacements in many stores.

- Cleanser, water, wipes — which to use? For newborn babies simple cotton wool and warm water is best. Most people decide to stop using these after a while and start using fragrance free wipes instead. Of course if you prefer to use the wipes straight away, do. Newborn babies have such perfect, delicate skin that you should avoid using fragranced wipes or soap as it will dehydrate the skin and leave it and more prone to infection and rash.
- Vaseline or Sudocrem? Vaseline (petroleum jelly) is a perfect barrier cream and helps prevent infection and soreness. If you do notice redness when you are changing the nappies then use the Sudocrem or similar medicated nappy rash ointment and it should clear up fairly quickly. As a rule of thumb I use Vaseline or similar petroleum jelly as a barrier cream for everyday use, and Sudocrem or similar nappy rash cream when little bums look red or sore.

## Disposable vs. Reusable Nappies

As with everything else, there is plenty of choice when it comes to buying nappies. Nappies are one of a handful of things that you will need lorry-loads of so it might be worth giving the topic a few moments thought. With at least eight or more nappy changes per baby per day in the beginning that's a lot of used nappies. So the main question is whether to dispose or not to dispose? Ultimately it's your choice and, as with every other choice you make concerning your babies, you should opt for what you believe is right and suits your family.

Disposable nappies have the advantage of being, well, for want of a better term, disposable. I was surviving on very little sleep and already had machine-loads of babygros to wash on top of everything else. I reckoned that if it saved a little bit of time and helped make this a bit easier then it was going to be disposables all the way for us. You're probably wondering why there is so much choice and discussion about different types of disposable nappies. I mean, they are all nappies, right? In the end it really comes down to a combination of your preference and what fits the babies best. You might find that some cheaper brands are not as strong as more expensive ones but as long as you change them often enough it shouldn't be too much of an issue.

Disposable nappies are quick and easy to change and if you have to change any while you are out and about you can bin the used ones and don't have to carry soiled nappies around in your bag all day until you get home. They are also relatively small so it's easy to pack a few into your changing bag. You can even buy special disposable swim-nappies for your baby to wear in the swimming pool.

Disposable nappies are not great for the environment though. The main alternative to these is reusable nappies. They are usually made of terry towelling or muslin and need to be washed, sterilised and dried after each use. The more you have, the less often you will use and wash each one, and the longer they will last. You will also need nappy liners, nappy pins, and plastic pants to put over the nappy. Nappy liners are placed inside the nappy and next to the babies' skin. They help reduce nappy rash and also help prevent the nappy from getting too badly soiled. Some fabric nappies have Velcro fasteners and are so easy to use that it's hard to see why they weren't around years ago. They speed up the process, are easy to use, and save you from stabbing your fingers with large nappy pins.

You might want to consider buying a dedicated wash basket or bin for the soiled nappies. This way you can keep the smelly soiled nappies away from the rest of your washing. A tumble dryer would also be handy as you will have a lot more laundry to get through. Tumble dryers are not so great for the environment though, so if you are using cloth nappies out of concern for a greener environment then the dryer will cancel out some of that good. Your increased laundry will mean that you do use more energy to run your washing machine more frequently. So, while you are not sending disposable nappies to landfill, you will be using more energy and increasing your carbon emissions.

The main advantage with reusable nappies is that they are a cheaper option over time. If you want to try them out there are lots of websites with advice on which ones to buy. You could also ask around amongst your friends to see whether any of them, or any of their friends or colleagues, have used them and can give you a few tips.

## BATHING

The word 'bath' used to conjure up images of luxurious, deep hot baths with scented candles, aromatic bath gels, and time to unwind and relax. After having twins the word 'bath' doesn't quite have the same effect! In the beginning it was a terrifying experience because one of the twins hated it and cried hysterically. After a while it got better but it was always a fairly labour intensive activity.

Bath time can also be a really special time. Once your twins get used to the bath it is lots of fun. It has so many benefits it really is worth sticking with it even if it is a screaming session at the start. Besides the obvious one which is that the babies will be nice and squeaky clean, it also helps them to relax and they should sleep better afterwards.

**Some tips to help with bath time:**

- The golden rule of bath time is to never leave the babies unsupervised. Don't take your hand or eyes off them, even for a second. Children can drown in less than an inch of water. If the phone rings don't worry, the caller will leave you a message and if it's important enough they will call you back later.
- Gather up all of the things you will need before you start.
- Make sure the room is warm enough before you start so the babies don't get cold when you take them out of the water.
- Run the water before you put either baby into the bath. It is better not to run the water while one of the babies is in the bath because the temperature can change too rapidly and you need both hands for the baby.
- The water should be a comfortable warm temperature. The nurses in the hospital teach you to test it with your elbow. You will soon get to know the right temperature with practice at home.
- Only put a few inches of water into the bath for your twins and no more than below waist high when your baby can sit up.
- Use lots of very soft, warm towels to help warm up, soothe and snuggle the babies afterwards.

- You can buy special bath mats for the twins to sit on in the bath once they can sit up by themselves to help prevent them slipping.
- Brightly coloured shapes stuck around the bath make the bath a bright and interesting fun place.
- If either of your babies' skin looks dry you can buy tubs of emollient cream to use as soap. It works wonders on dry skin but is fairly greasy when it hits the water so just make sure you have a good grip on the baby with one arm before you apply the cream with the other. It's a bit of an art but being a mother of twins you'll be able to master it in no time.

That's all fine when the babies are either a few months old and don't roll around the bathroom banging into everything so you can bath them one at a time, or they are old enough to sit up by themselves and can go into the bath together. There is an awkward period in between when the babies are crawling and are not big enough to go into the bath together and won't lie still on the floor if you bath them one at a time. I sometimes brought a bouncing chair into the bathroom at this stage and took turns putting one baby into the chair with toys and one baby into the bath. I'd love to tell you that this is the perfect solution that works like a charm all of the time but in reality there was always someone who didn't want to go into the chair! This is when help comes in really handy. If you have someone to help you, you can let them play with whichever baby is not in the bath.

## CRYING

Every parent struggles with this one, especially in the beginning. It can be even more difficult to cope with when you have twins who are crying in stereo. The thing is though, crying is totally normal. If you can expect it and somehow manage to accept it and treat it as normal, then you will find it easier to cope with. It's your babies' only real method of communicating with you and expressing feelings of cold or hunger or consternation at being left alone for too long. The twins need to have some way to tell you if they are hungry or their nappy needs to be changed. I do feel a little hypocritical saying that as I found the twins crying upsetting in the beginning. There were days when I felt like I had done a full day's work by 9am and those usually featured both twins crying together at some stage or other before I had even got dressed.

Don't be afraid of spoiling the babies by picking them up. Yes, it is important for them to learn to fall asleep by themselves and to be able to spend time in their cots awake and alone. But when they are so small it is perfectly fine to pick them up and enjoy lots of cuddles while you can. You are not spoiling them. You are bonding with them and they are learning that you are there for them and will respond to them when they need you.

The main thing to remember when the babies are crying is that it is completely normal. All babies cry and if yours don't then maybe you should consider having a chat with your local doctor or district nurse about it. All babies cry for lots of reasons and you can often figure out the reason for the tears through a process of elimination. Work your way through the list and see what you're left with.

## Crying for Food

This is normally the easiest one to deal with. Unless both twins wake up and start crying for a feed at the same time. I found myself in some hilarious contortions trying to feed two newborns at the same time. Talk about multi-tasking! The key to surviving it is to be organised. If you are bottle feeding have all of your bottles prepared and the milk powder measured out in specially designed powder holders and ready to go. If you are breast feeding you have less preparation to do but still need to make sure you are looking after yourself and eating enough when you can. Keep lots of bibs and wipes beside where you usually do your feeding so that when it all goes pear-shaped you won't have to pull the house apart in a panic looking for a bib or cloth when both twins are wailing louder than a siren for food at the same time.

I'm sure you will have realised by now how many conflicting ideas there are about when you should feed your baby. Normally in hospital you are advised to feed approximately every three hours. If one baby is having difficulty taking in enough at a time then you might be advised to give them a feed every two hours. Babies don't really stick to clocks though, so if one baby is looking for a feed half an hour early then go with it and give the feed when they need it, especially in those early weeks. Tiny babies need to feed as often as they want to gain weight and stay hydrated. As time goes by you will need to start getting them into a more regular pattern so that you can start to establish a routine. In those first few weeks home from hospital though you should feed the babies when they need it. The babies are learning how to take in a feed and learning to tell you when they need more by having a good cry. They are also learning that you will respond to this most basic need and feed them when they need it. So they are learning to trust you and developing a relationship with you already.

## Crying because of Wind

Babies need help to bring up wind after every feed and there are few things as painful as trapped wind. I think I spent as much time winding the babies as I did feeding them or doing anything else. It does get a bit tedious after a while but stick with it. It's nice to have a baby on your shoulder while you rub their back and it's a great excuse for a little cuddle.

## Crying with Colic

Colic is often the cause when babies cry for long periods at a time each day for a few weeks or more for no obvious reason[10]. It normally starts when the babies are a few weeks old and ends within three to five months. It often starts with crying in the afternoon; our twins cried from 3pm until 5 or 6 pm every day when they had it. Sometimes the babies pull their knees up their chest as if they are in pain and it can be very difficult to find a comfortable position for them. It can be very hard to deal with especially when you are only getting a couple of hours sleep each night.

It also doesn't help that you have two babies to deal with and if both have colic you'll really be stretched to your limit. Remember it's not your fault; you are doing a great job. Also remember it won't last forever and it will definitely get easier. It doesn't get harder than what you are going through now. If your friends or family offer to help get them to call around during the colic hours so that they can help carry the babies around or rub their backs or tummies or whatever you want them to do to help.

In most cases the babies just grow out of it after a few months. This might be bad news on one hand because now you know this might be something that you are going to have to suffer through for a few months. On the other hand take heart, it is good news because it will come to an end and won't last forever. There are various drops and remedies you can buy to add to your babies bottle to help lessen the symptoms.

So when is the crying from colic, and when is it something else more serious? Sometimes babies have difficulties digesting lactose (the sugars in milk). Symptoms include crying, diarrhoea, vomiting, and eczema. If your baby cries after feeding, vomits it all back up, and seems to be suffering from trapped wind and diarrhoea then chances are they are suffering from this. Don't confuse it with colic; the symptoms are much more severe. Talk to your doctor to confirm your suspicions and see how to go about treating it. They may suggest trying a soya-based substitute or it might take a trip to a paediatrician who will prescribe special milk for your babies.

## Crying for a Nappy Change

Some babies find it more uncomfortable than others to have a nappy that needs to be changed and they will certainly let you know all about it. Others really don't like having their nappies changed and will cry as soon as you lay them down on the changing mat. Try chatting and singing and have toys and brightly coloured shapes nearby to make nappy changing a fun time.

## Crying for Attention and Entertainment

Of course your twins might be crying because they are just plain old bored! Their different personalities will be a factor in this. Are they content to lie on a mat and watch you clean or cook or get on with your list of jobs, or watch their twin brother or sister play with their hands or feet, or the sunlight make shapes on the walls? If not, and they would rather have your attention and be carried around by you, then they are more likely to cry when you put them down.

Some babies are just not content to watch shadows and shapes, they want to be entertained and they want it now. Even most adults would be bored if they had to sit in one placed for any length of time with no-one to talk to and nothing to amuse them. So, if your babies are well fed and winded and nappies recently changed, no pains or aches and are not tired, but are still crying — then it's a good bet that they are a bit bored. Nothing a few songs and toys won't sort!

## Crying for Peace and Quiet

On the other hand, if it's been a busy and noisy few hours then it is quite likely that the babies will start crying for a bit of peace and quiet. I can relate to that too! Newborn babies are used to hearing the sound of your heartbeat and your voice and very little other stimulation. Then suddenly they are born and have to deal with a whole range of lights, sounds, and action and it can all get a bit much. Babies experience this daily in the beginning as they get used to the sensations of sound and vision. They grow out of it as they get bigger and more used to everything. Tiredness definitely plays a role in this too. As they start to spend any amount of time awake they also get more tired and by late afternoon they are overtired and overloaded.

There are a few practical things you can do to help calm things down and restore some peace:

- Take the babies into a darkened and quiet room. If they are over-stimulated then it makes sense to remove some of the lights and sounds.
- Swaddle the babies tightly in snug blankets (or sheets if your house is warm). Babies love the security of being swaddled. Being tightly wrapped also prevents them from squirming too much and helps them to relax.
- If anyone offers to help you get them to call during the 'crying hour' so they can hold, feed, or soothe, one of the babies for you.

# Feeding your Twins

## TO BREASTFEED OR TO BOTTLE FEED?

This is the big question. Along with routines and sleeping through the night, the issue of whether to breastfeed or bottle feed is one of the hottest topics for discussion when it comes to new baby care. Everyone has advice of course and not all of it good. All you can do is to find out what is best for you and your troupe and stick to that.

### Breast Feeding

There are some well-documented advantages to breastfeeding. There are also some myths, some scares, and some painful things to watch out for and avoid, or at least treat as quickly as you can. The nursing staff in the hospital should be only too happy to show you how to get the babies to 'latch on' correctly and will be there to help you as often as you need. Take this time to get as much advice and help as you can so that when you get home you are as confident as you can be that you are doing things correctly. There are breast-feeding support groups that you can join, or even just contact should you need advice.

It can take a few days for your milk supply to come in properly, so if you find that the babies are getting hysterical in those first two or three days, it may be the case that they are simply just hungry. I know people who have given their babies a bottle in the middle of the night at this stage, just to keep them fed and happy. All of the professional advice is to stick with breastfeeding if you choose this method. However, it is important to be realistic and sometimes you have to just go with it and give the babies a bottle if that is what they need most at that time.

It can also be very confusing trying to figure out how long you should feed each baby for. A friend said she was told by a nurse to feed her baby for ten minutes on each side. She followed this advice to the letter, only to find that her baby was hungry and cried a lot. You are the twins' mum and you are the person to gauge best how hungry the babies are and how much they need to feed. If they are hungry and need more, then that's fine. On the other hand, if they don't seem hungry that day, then that's fine too. Monitor their intake over a couple of days or a week instead of just one day to get a better picture of whether they are feeding enough.

*The Benefits*

- During the first three days after the babies are born the breasts produce colostrum that will help your babies stay healthy and strong. This is a mix of water, protein and minerals and contains antibodies. These antibodies help to prevent infections and also help to protect the babies' intestine from bacteria.
- Breastfeeding is more convenient than bottle-feeding because you don't have to spend time messing about with sterilisers (unless, of course, you wish to express). If you are breastfeeding you can head out with your gang without having to spend the morning making bottles and measuring formula into powder holders. You will still need to pack wipes and cloths but will save so much time by not having to prepare bottles in advance. It means you can be more spontaneous too because preparing bottles requires timing and planning.
- A lot of people believe that breastfeeding can help you to lose weight. Breastfeeding produces oxytocin, which in turn prompts the uterus to shrink[11]. You do have to eat regularly though to help your body produce the extra milk you need.

Just watch that you are filling up on healthy food rather than treats or before you know it you'll have developed a fondness for chocolate chip cookies that stays with you long after the twins have stopped breastfeeding and you have gained more weight than you lost.

## Myths & Scares

Ovulation is often limited while breastfeeding[12], causing many people to believe that you can't get pregnant while breastfeeding. This is not always the case, so don't depend on it. While ovulation may have been suppressed, it has not been stopped altogether and we all know a few people who have had a little surprise a few months after one baby was born. After having twins it is advisable to talk to your doctor about your options, particularly if you have had a Caesarean Section.

Many people worry that their babies will choke while they are breastfeeding and this is a very normal concern. Babies are able to swallow when they are born so they won't choke. If you are concerned that your milk is flowing too quickly simply express some milk first before you start.

## Painful Issues

Unfortunately there can be some downsides to breastfeeding and occasionally you might experience cracked nipples, painful engorgement, or blocked ducts. The best way to avoid these is to make sure your twins are latching on properly and feed your babies regularly. Look after yourself well and keep your breasts dry in between feeds. Wear a bra that fits correctly and loose fitting clothes.

More serious painful complaints such as mastitis or breast abscesses will require making a visit to your G.P. and you will probably need some antibiotics to clear up the infection.

## How does it Work with Twins?!

So that's all fine if you are just trying to learn how to breastfeed one baby but what happens when you have twins? It is possible to breastfeed both babies at the same time and many people have managed successfully. They all say it takes dedication and determination and it is perfectly normal to worry about low milk supply, whether the babies are feeding enough, and whether you'll ever have a break.

**Here are a few tips from mums who have been there:**

- Find out as much as you can before the twins arrive to help you prepare mentally and in practical ways too.
- Get all the help you can from the staff in the hospital. Ask them every question you can think of and keep asking until you are happy that you are getting the hang of it.
- Buy nursing cushions. There are some specially designed ones for feeding twins. These enable you to feed both twins together quite comfortably.
- Buy very comfortable nursing bras.
- If you are worried that you are not producing enough milk then simply just feed more often. The more the babies feed the more milk you will produce.
- Feeding two babies should not hurt more than feeding one baby at a time. If the twins have latched on correctly then you shouldn't be sore.
- Feed the babies as often as they need it. Ignore anyone who is telling you to get them into a routine in the beginning and just go with the flow. With two babies to manage you will all benefit if you eliminate stress.
- Keep eating.
- Drink lots of water.
- You can take a break. You can express some milk so that the babies can have a bottle from time to time and you can get someone else to feed them while you head out for a walk or a have soak in the bath, or even just sleep.
- Join your local La Leche League or other local Breastfeeding Association for help and support.
- Lots of people say that breastfeeding gets easier after three months when the twins get bigger and faster at taking a feed.
- Go online and read blogs and articles written by mums of twins who have breastfed their babies. Their stories and advice will not only help you figure out how to feed your

own twins, their stories and experiences will give you a boost and encourage you that you are not alone in this and that you will get through it.

- Don't feel guilty about stopping when the time is right for you. The most important thing is that your babies are feeding well, and if you managed to breastfeed them at all then you deserve a medal and should be proud of your achievement.

There are some scary urban myths out there about the super-mom who always managed to breastfeed both twins at the same time, all of the time. While it is certainly possible to breastfeed both babies at the same time, don't feel pressurised by the stories. If you manage to breastfeed the twins at all you will be doing very well. Give yourself a break and don't listen to these stories so early on. There are 'wonder-woman' stories out there about every single aspect of raising kids. If you start listening to them now, and feeling under pressure to perform, you will only set yourself up to feel more inadequate later on. Do the best you can, and don't be too hard on yourself. Half of the stories are probably exaggerated anyway.

## Bottle Feeding

Breastfeeding isn't always an option, or the only option. I chose bottle feeding for my twins and was able to accept lots of help in the early days, much as it pained me to ask for it. Having twins by Caesarean Section meant that I simply could not do everything myself, which would be my normal instinct. Instead, I had to rope in our families to help with bottle feeds and everything else.

One of the big advantages of bottle feeding is that the twins' dad can be just as involved with the babies as you are. Breastfeeding excludes everyone else, but sometimes the dads want to be able to give feeds too. Bottle-feeding is an easy way to spend time with your new twins and bond with them and it's great for the fathers to be able to do this. With twins there are so many feeds a day that having someone else to help is only ever an advantage. On average, new babies tend to take a bottle once every two to three hours. That means a minimum of eight bottles per day per baby, 16 bottles in total on a very good day and up to twenty on a more normal one. I spent the days and nights calculating maths computations that wouldn't be out of place on an exam paper:

*Both babies take 1 hour to feed, wind and change nappies and you want to feed them one at a time. Twin 1 was last fed at 2 o'clock. The time now is 3.45. At what time should you feed twin 2 in order to keep some time free for sterilising and laundry?*

Complicated? Absolutely! Especially at 4.30 in the morning when I'd been in bed for an hour and knew that the next time I got out of bed I'd be up for the day. I'd hear one of the babies start to make their little pre-waking snuffling sounds and start calculating again: if I stay in bed for another half an hour, does it leave enough time to feed twin 2 before twin 1 wakes up again, or should I just pick twin 2 up now to be sure of having enough time to feed each one on their own? Thankfully this phase doesn't last too long.

Bottle feeding may be your best option for other reasons besides enlisting family members to help with feeds. Physically you may not be able to manage it. There is no shame in that at all and it is more common than you think.

One of my twins had a bit of difficulty getting the hang of drinking and swallowing in the beginning and would take ages to drink the smallest amounts. Bottle feeding meant that my husband or whoever was helping could sit with him for as long as he needed while I fed the other twin and got on with things. Bottle feeding him meant that I could see exactly what quantity he was actually taking in at each sitting.

---

**DID YOU KNOW?**
*Bottle-fed babies can get little lip blisters in the beginning. These are harmless and will heal up quickly*

---

## Milk Formula

There are several different milk formula options available. Most basic milk formulas are pretty similar; it's really up to you which one you choose. Your doctor may advise a special formula if you feel the basic ones are causing problems. Don't switch formula without consulting your doctor first.

You can buy formula in powder form or in ready-made cartons. Powder lasts longer and is less expensive than ready-made formula. On the other hand, ready-made formula is quick and handy when you are under pressure for time during those first few weeks home from the hospital. Follow the guidelines on the packaging and never use milk leftover from an earlier feed.

## Preparing Feeds

Boil a kettle of water and leave to cool for thirty minutes. When cooled, pour into sterilised bottles. Fill each bottle with the amount you will need for a single feed for one baby and add the correct amount of formula for the amount of water in the bottle. There is no need to chill or heat the bottle as long as you have sterilised the bottles and used boiled water.

## The Golden Rules

There are a few golden rules to remember when bottle feeding:

---

**DO**
- *Wash your hands first before doing anything.*
- *Sterilise everything.*
- *Make up the bottles strictly according to the instructions on the tin.*
- *Add the formula when you need a bottle.*
- *Give more if the twins need it.*

**DON'T**
- *Don't leave your twins to take a bottle propped up on their own with a cushion as they could choke.*
- *Don't be tempted to add in a bit of extra formula.*
- *Don't use leftover bottles later on. Any milk left at the end of the feed should be thrown out straight away.*
- *Don't heat the milk in a microwave as it doesn't heat the bottle evenly.*

---

- Don't worry if your twins don't finish a bottle.
- If the bottle is too hot don't be tempted to top it up with cold water from the tap. Don't laugh; this actually happens! Always use cooled boiled water to make up the bottles and if they are too hot simply cool under a cold tap or stand in a jug of cold water.

## BY THE CLOCK VS. ON-DEMAND FEEDING

There are two fairly differing schools of thought on how to approach feeding. One school advocates feeding 'on-demand'. With this method the babies should be fed whenever they need and as often as they need. The babies choose when they want to be fed. This is very relaxed for everyone as you aren't trying to keep track of times and babies aren't crying for feeds. Your babies are learning that you will answer them when they need something. It is limiting though, as your schedule will be more unpredictable and you may end up feeding quite frequently, which will leave you less time for other things. Interestingly, the American Association of Paediatrics is strongly in favour of on-demand feeding[13].

The other school advocates feeding strictly according to the clock. As far as possible, the babies should be fed at certain times. Eventually they should start to anticipate their feeds and settle into the routine. This gives structure to your day and helps create time for you and the babies apart from feeds.

So which to choose? I know people who fed their babies according to both methods and both seemed to get along fine with the system they chose. I do suspect that these friends chose the methods which best suited their personality, I would have been a lot more surprised had either chosen the other way instead. I tended to take a more pragmatic approach to feeding. Babies are just like adults; their appetites vary from feed to feed, and from day to day. If the babies are crying and are clearly hungry, why let them (and you and everyone else in the house) suffer? So I tried to keep to regular feed times as much as was practical. However, if the babies were having a hungry day I went with it and fed more as needed. Similarly, if the twins left a bit behind in their bottles, that was ok too. Very quickly the babies fell into their own natural patterns anyway (see Chapter 6 for more on routines). As the months went by, they were able to take more in each feed and the time in between feeds naturally stretched out to regular bottle times.

If you want to feed them both at the same time you might consider letting the hungrier baby set the feeding times.

> *After having experienced the sleep-deprived craziness of a minimum of 16 feeds a day I can honestly say it gets easier!*
>
> *As the twins grow bigger they can take more in each bottle and need fewer feeds. Hang in there, it will get easier soon!*

## MORE FEEDING KNOW-HOW

### Baby Diary

I had often heard other mums talking about 'baby brain' and I definitely had a case of it during those early months of sleep deprivation. I could never remember what time the twins had taken their last bottle, how much of their bottles they had managed to take, or whether the nappies were wet or dirty. It turns out that tracking babies' nappies can reveal a lot about their health at that time. For example, a decrease in the number of wet nappies can indicate that the babies are not drinking enough, or a lack of dirty nappies can show up constipation. When all of these details are written down you may spot a trend earlier than you would do otherwise.

So, crazy as it sounds, we kept a diary listing all the feeds and nappy changes from the day. It gave us peace of mind at the time to be able to see how much the twins had taken in their bottles over the day. I'm sure this is something a second-time mum wouldn't bother with but as an exhausted first-timer with a brain like a sieve I found it useful. It also gives you a written record of the twins' feeds over the week so you see at a glance whether they are feeding enough.

## SAMPLE BABY DIARY

| Day | Feed Amount Twin A | Nappy Twin A | Feed Amount Twin B | Nappy Twin B |
|---|---|---|---|---|
| Time | | | | |
| Time | | | | |
| Time | | | | |
| Time | | | | |

## Sterilising

Why do you need to sterilise everything anyway? Sterilising gets rid of harmful bacteria that can cause illness, so bottles, bottle tops and teats should be sterilised after each use. The best approach is to wash all bottles and feeding equipment thoroughly as soon as possible after a feed before any leftover milk can dry and stick to awkward corners. Don't forget to include the scoop that comes with the milk formula or the tongs for the steriliser.

There are lots of different ways to sterilise bottles. By far the easiest way is to buy sterilising equipment which will do the job for you. With twins you will need to sterilise so many bottles that a steriliser can be a lifesaver. There are many different methods of sterilising to suit every preference and budget (see Chapter 2 for more information on the different types of sterilisers available).

Take care when opening your steriliser lid as the steam can be very hot. Whichever method you choose, make sure to follow the manufacturer's instructions carefully.

## Winding

After each feed you should gently 'wind' your babies. Babies are not able to bring up wind on their own because their muscles and reflexes are still developing. Sit your baby on your knee supporting them with one hand on their front while you gently rub their back with your other hand. Alternatively, you can place the baby on your shoulder and gently rub their back. Don't pat them too hard and remember to cover your knees or back with a cloth as babies can often spit back some of the feed when they burp.

## MOVING ONTO SOLIDS

This is an enormous milestone. It is exciting and fun but it can also be daunting and difficult to know when to move on to this stage. As a general rule, if your twins are not sleeping at night for as long as they had been and you feel that their normal feed is not filling them up, they are probably ready for solid food. Official guidelines say to start at six months but in reality most people start a month earlier.

A lot of books recommend starting out with fruit. However, a friend of mine suggested a great tip which was to start with baby rice and vegetables for a week or two. That way the babies won't develop an early sweet tooth and prefer fruit to vegetables. Baby rice is great and you can mix pureed vegetables or pureed fruit with it. Keep it simple with one meal of baby rice per day for the first week to let your twins get the hang of eating and digesting food.

Try new fruits or vegetables one at a time. It's good to let babies get to taste things individually. Introduce new foods early in the day and give them the same thing for a few days to see how they get on with it. You will soon spot whether the new food is having any strange effects.

There is no need to add sugar or salt. Babies' kidneys are not sufficiently developed to cope with too much salt so never add it. Fruits contain natural sugars and some vegetables are sweet tasting too. If you add sugar you will encourage your twins to develop a sweet-tooth and harm their gums and baby teeth.

It is much cheaper to prepare your own babies' meals than to buy them. It is time-consuming though. The good news is that you can cook in batches and freeze all of it in small containers.

There are some excellent baby recipe books available and I highly recommend investing in one. Books such as Annabel Karmel's 'New Complete Baby and Toddler Meal Planner' (Ebury Press, 2007) guide you through menus for babies at this fairly tricky stage.

It will help you to introduce the right foods at the right time and ensure lots of variety. It is all too easy to fall into a habit of making the same couple of meals over and over again. Following a baby meal plan helps avoid falling into that trap. (See also Appendix 2 for some recipe ideas for hungry babies).

---

**TOP TIPS**

- *Start with vegetables to avoid babies preferring sweet things*
- *Cook in batches and freeze the extra portions*
- *Let your twins experiment with feeding themselves. The mess is worth it if they learn to feed themselves and eat well*
- *Follow a meal plan to ensure lots of variety*
- *Avoid cow's milk, honey, pate, soft cheese and nuts until the twins are over one year old*

---

## Whether to Feed Separately or Together

In the beginning, when our twins were tiny, I used to try to feed them individually because they were bottle fed and I found it very difficult to hold both babies and both bottles at the same time. Obviously things didn't always go to plan and I would end up with two babies screaming to be fed together. Of course it is possible to bottle-feed both babies at the same time. I discovered afterwards that those specially designed cushions for breastfeeding can also be adapted for bottle feeding. All you need is the shaped cushions and some creativity; just don't leave the babies all alone with a bottle.

When the twins got much bigger and could sit up on their own they were more content to be bottle-fed at the same time in their high chairs and even started trying to hold the bottle themselves. It didn't happen overnight, just a gradual transition. Once the twins were happy with this arrangement I often fed them this way instead. It did free up a lot of time, which I was grateful for. So, when it came to starting the twins on solid food I was able to feed them both at the same time. There are so many advantages to this. The overriding benefit is the time gained. When you first start the babies on solids you will still be feeding them milk, so if you were to do all of these feeds individually you would never have time to do anything else all day. You can just make one batch of food to feed both babies which saves time at every stage of the feed, from preparing the food to feeding and cleaning up afterwards.

## FREEZING FOOD

Babies eat such tiny portions that you will usually have enough food leftover to freeze for another day. Ideally try to cook in bigger batches so that you can freeze plenty of portions and therefore cut down on your cooking time.

There are a few food safety rules to keep in mind when freezing food:

- Leave a little space at the top of the container because the frozen food will expand slightly.
- Freeze meals in the correct portion sizes so that you can just defrost the amount you want at a time.
- Chill food before you freeze it.
- Don't re-freeze anything once it has been defrosted.
- Trust your nose and your eyes. If something looks a bit dodgy after it has been defrosted just throw it out.
- If there is a power cut don't open the freezer door. Your frozen food should be fine for up to 24 hours as long as the freezer door remains shut [14].
- Label everything because you won't remember what everything is five minutes after you have put the pots into the fridge.

Most of the meals you cook can be frozen; however, some foods do not freeze well such as cooked eggs, potatoes (mashed potatoes are fine), cream, salads and raw vegetables. Finally, there are some surprising things that do freeze well. Milk will freeze for a month, butter and margarine and most bread will keep for up to three months. Grated cheese can be frozen too and you can add it to your cooking straightaway without having to defrost it first.

# 6

# The Great Routine Debate

## ROUTINES – WHAT'S THE BIG FUSS?

So much has been written on this subject and everyone has an opinion on the matter. Even total strangers will ask you whether your twins are in a routine simply for something to say. It can feel like a fairly competitive area too. You will be told stories about babies that sleep through the night at four weeks old. These are the same babies that can walk and talk at ten months so it's good to learn not to pay too much attention to these tall tales or you will end up feeling stressed and inferior, and worrying about your twins' perfectly normal development for absolutely no good reason.

So what is a 'routine' anyway? It simply just means getting a system going. Babies **do** like some form of routine. They like to have clear boundaries and a predictable pattern to the day. They like to have some form of a bedtime ritual. Knowing what to expect makes them feel safe and secure.

There are a few different approaches to establishing a routine, much like the different approaches to feeding. 'Parent-led' routines are based around a timetable determined by the parents. This method follows the clock and is designed to be structured and organised similar to 'by-the-clock' feeding schedules. Followers of this routine like the control and order of a strict timetable. There are many books out there with suggested timetables and strategies to help you get up and running if this sounds like it would suit you. These routines are controversial because there is a risk that you will ignore your twins' signs of hunger and they will not feed enough. If the twins do not feed enough there is a risk that they won't gain enough weight and will become dehydrated.

'Baby-led' routines are dictated by the babies own natural patterns. It can be very flexible and sometimes a little disorganised. Followers of this type of routine take all of their cues from the baby and allow their needs and wants to dictate the day. Feeds happen when the twins are hungry, i.e. on-demand, but never more than four hours apart. Playtime and naptime also happen whenever the twins seem ready for them. This means that the twins will more than likely take their feeds and have a nap at a different time every day. The main advantage of this type of routine is that nobody gets stressed while trying to fit things in at prescribed times. Disadvantages include a lack of time for yourself or anyone else, and a lack of predictability. It can also be difficult to leave your twins alone with anyone else because they will not be able to read their little signs as well as you can and won't know what their cries mean or what to do next.

Thirdly, there are the somewhere-in-between routines which take the best points of both and are moulded to fit your family and you. Whichever you choose, the twins' wellbeing is most important. Books written about 'combination' routines advocate sticking to a pattern of feeding, playing and napping in that order, but not worrying about the time. They have all the advantages of a routine that anyone can follow without any of the stress of keeping to a rigid timetable. While the twins are still newborn babies you should always feed them when they seem hungry, even if they were fed in the last hour or two, to make sure they are gaining the correct weight and staying hydrated. Similarly, if they are not hungry don't force them to finish a feed as they will spit it all back up later.

Whatever customs and habits you put in place that suit your baby and fit well into your daily schedule will work just fine. Just try to stick to it. Babies love and need consistency of care, so as long as you try to stick to your routine as much as possible then you will all reap the benefits. Occasionally your twins may get sick after you have worked so hard to get them into a lovely smooth routine and all of your hard work goes out of the window. You just have to start all over again when they recover.

## ROUTINES AND TWINS

How does any routine work with twins? I decided to view it as a pattern to the day, a sequence of tasks fitted into a time frame that would ultimately make the day flow more easily. I kept our baby diary beside all of the baby gear and noted down their feed times and quantities. Having the information written down made it much easier to see the twins' own natural patterns start to become apparent. We were able to use this information to establish our schedule.

After a few months we settled into our own system, and you will too. We combined the structure of parent-led routines with the flexibility of baby-led routines. In other words, the activities remained the same but didn't necessarily happen at exactly the same time every day. If someone was having a hungry day they fed more and got through the process more quickly and more often.

Our system was based on the 'combination routines' style and would involve a nappy change, a bottle, some activity time and a nap. I then used some of the nap time for chores and the rest of the nap time to sit down and switch off. As the twins got bigger they grew easier to manage together at the same time which meant that I started to be able to get them into their cots for a sleep at the same time and I got a break. I could also start to predict times for activities and plan to get us all out for walks or visits to friends and relatives.

Having a system means that everyone knows what is happening and you are less likely to forget to do something important like sterilise bottles in time. The babies get used to doing things in sequence too and are less stressed. They learn to anticipate the next event in the sequence. I am still convinced that this helped them to stretch out the time in between feeds particularly at night time.

Another advantage of having your own system like this is that it takes the stress out of your twins crying. If you know your twins have been fed, winded, and had their nappy changed and they are still crying you know you don't need to waste lots of time trying to feed them more when they don't need it. My twins used to have a 'crying time' every day. I think they just needed to release a bit of steam after the build up from all the noise and routine of the day. I was able to arrange to have help during this crying time from friends and family a lot of days in the beginning to help with it.

## TIPS FOR A SUCCESSFUL ROUTINE

1. **Keep it simple**. Like most things in life, the simpler you keep it, the more likely you are to succeed. Routines are no different. If you over-complicate things you will lose track and forget what happens next, and completely stress yourself out in the process. Not to mention your partner, your family, the twins and anyone else within a two-mile radius. No-one will be able to keep up and you will all end up wanting to cry more often than you should or would do otherwise. Overly complicated routines defeat the purpose of having one in the first place. Instead, keep it all nice and simple.

2. **Use your Baby Diary to get started**. The great advantage of keeping a diary like this is that you can begin to see a pattern emerge as the twins grow bigger. You can use this information as a starting point for your routine.

3. **Build in a regular nappy change time**, always excepting any emergency changes of course. You know the ones when that unmistakeable smell suddenly fills the room! Otherwise a regular nappy changing time is good and helps you focus your time instead of losing time checking nappies that didn't need to be changed, or forget to change them altogether.

4. **Build in a regular feeding time.** This is difficult in the beginning, especially if you are breastfeeding. Of course, if the babies are obviously hungry then you should feed them. It helps to try to keep the feed in the same sequence each time when you can.

5. **Build in playtime**. Babies learn by playing and exploring.

6. **Build in time for chores.** Nothing helps you feel back in control like having a few of the jobs ticked off the list, whether it's having the washing machine switched on or the bottles washed and sterilised. I used to spend some time after both babies were fed, winded and changed to try and get washing into the machine, or out of it and into the dryer, or potatoes peeled or something. I also used to clear the kitchen worktops so that when the next round of feed-winding-nappies started I could look around and see order and feel some sense of achievement.

7. **Build in time for you.** It's too easy to spend the precious time between the babies finally going to sleep and the first one waking back up again for a feed on jobs and chores. Prioritise your chores and make sure you take ten minutes out for yourself. Put the kettle on, have a shower, or read a few pages of a book. It will help keep you sane! There will always be jobs to do; there will not always be time for you to sit down for a few minutes rest on your own.

8. **Be consistent** — Babies like consistency as much as adults do. If you have a regular pattern to your day your babies will start to anticipate what's happening next, and they will be more relaxed. You will be more relaxed because you will have time to get a few things done and a cup of tea to yourself. Now it wouldn't be entirely accurate to suggest that life will be plain sailing once you have your routine established! There are days when the babies are cranky and for reasons unknown the day turns into a bit of a disaster and any attempt at routine goes right out the window. It can start with the smallest thing, like a horrific nappy and suddenly you are in the middle of a fiasco with two screaming, and hungry babies who both need to be fed, winded and changed again, while unsterilised bottles and laundry pile up. But the good news is that those days happen less often as time goes by.

9. **Be flexible.** This does not contradict consistency. Routines are so important and will help you in so many ways. However, it's good not to be too rigid about it. While it is important to have a certain amount of consistency and structure in your day, it's okay too to do something differently some days. Don't miss out on days out or visits to friends and grandparents etc just because it means feeding the babies at a different time, or them sleeping in the car instead of their cribs or cots. Sometimes a small change or a day out can freshen everything up.

10. **Be realistic.** The fact is, that with two small babies to look after all day long, you simply will not have time to wash all of the windows, dust behind the radiators, or clean out the attic. Be realistic about what you can achieve — you may have to lower your expectations to do this. You will be less stressed and your entire family will thank you for it.

11. **Don't give in to competition**. For first-time mums who are unsure about so much it's very easy to feel inadequate when you hear some of the amazing stories you hear about other people's incredibly ordered and easy life. It's best to try not to pay too much attention to these! Unless your babies are really missing their milestones by a long way, then rest assured that you are doing a fine job and just because they still need a feed during the night, you are not a failure. Regular visits to your public health nurse will keep both your babies assessed for all of these things and your mind at ease. Remember, you are the babies' mum; you are the person who knows best how they are doing.

12. **Do what works for you**. There are umpteen books written on the subject and more conflicting advice than you could know what to do with. Remember that you have devised your routine for your family taking into account what works for you all. Stick to your guns and don't feel under pressure to change things simply because someone else thinks something different.

13. **Be prepared to change it as the babies grow**. As the twins develop their needs change so what works at one stage won't work so well at another. You won't have any problems as long as you keep this in mind and simply adapt your systems to their needs as you go along.

## BEDTIME

With the twins settling into a system of daytime feeds I began to treat the last daytime feed as a bedtime one. I started a 'bedtime routine' even though the twins still needed to be fed during the night. I reckoned that if I started a bedtime routine while they were still babies this would be well established by the time they were old enough to understand what was happening. So I used to change their nappies and get them ready for bed just before the last bottle around 7 o'clock. As the twins got a bit bigger we would read a little story at this time instead of having a 'playtime'. This meant they were sitting quietly and calmly enough to be put into their cots for bed. Having a bedtime routine had a great side effect that was very welcome and which we still enjoy today; the kids go to bed around 7ish and we get to enjoy an evening together, or have time for hobbies or to go to the gym etc.

Of course it took a long time to get this working like clockwork and there were many evenings when things really did not go to plan at all. If the twins were sick or out of sorts or even hyper our evening was spent trotting up and down the stairs. When the twins were small they liked to have our company while they fell asleep. But they could take over an hour to go to sleep and the evening would slip away while we sat and waited for them to nod off. Every child is different and when the twins were around a year old we ended up using two different approaches to break this habit of having to stay in the room for hours while the twins went to sleep. With my daughter we took the short-sharp-crying approach which meant having to endure her crying for a short while. The first night I said goodnight and left her she cried for forty minutes before she nodded off. I stood outside her door watching to make sure she was alright and kept checking on her so she knew I hadn't abandoned her; I just wanted her to learn to fall asleep by herself. The next night she cried for just under half an hour and the night after ten minutes. After only a few days we were able to leave her to go to sleep by herself. With my son I took a slightly different approach in the end as the crying one wasn't working as well for him. Over a period of time I cut five minutes off the amount of time I spent in the room with him. He got used to falling asleep on his own without really noticing it. Eventually I was just able to say goodnight and leave and he would play with his teddies and drop off to sleep on his own.

Every child is different and every parent is different and you can decide for yourself whether the short sharp approach with a bit of crying will work, or whether the longer, more subtle approach will work for you better. Either way it is well worth doing. Having a quiet evening together when the babies are asleep is so important. It gives you time to catch up on each other's news and relax together. It frees up a bit of time to get out for a walk or pop to the gym. It also gives you time to have an evening meal together so at least you know you will have one good meal each day. Best of all it means that a bedtime routine has been established from the beginning and you don't have the difficulty of introducing one to wary and reluctant toddlers later on. If they have had free reign during the evenings for as long as they can remember, they will naturally resist any sort of more formal routine being imposed. Most importantly, it means that your twins will be getting the full amount of sleep that they need.

## SAMPLE ROUTINE

This very simple routine works well and includes all of the most important activities: feeding and changing nappies as well as playtime and naptime for the twins and time for chores and a rest for you. We followed a pattern like this and found it very simple and easy to follow as well as being flexible enough to adapt as we went along.

## DAYTIME:

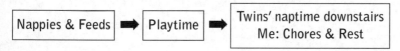

This daytime pattern of nappies-feeds-playtime-nap was repeated several times throughout the day as necessary.

## EVENING:

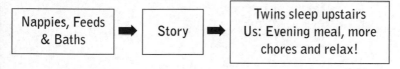

The last daytime feed around 7pm was followed by a story time instead of a playtime. We the put the twins to bed upstairs in their cots instead of letting them nap downstairs.

## NIGHT-TIME

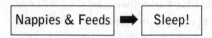

During the night we tried to keep feeds as simple as possible with a nappy change and a bottle and as little other time spent out of bed as we could get away with. With twins that still adds up to a lot of time spent awake during the night so the more you do to help yourself get some more seep the better! It does get easier as the twins begin to grasp the concepts of day and night and figure out that playtime only happens during the day.

# 7

# After the Storm

So you have survived the crazy early weeks and are starting to get used to having two newborn babies and all the demands, tears, laughs, and sleep deprivation that goes with that. Your friends may have said to you that things improve after six weeks, others may be more realistic and honest and say twelve weeks, and that's largely true. In reality, with twins, time passes and things become more familiar and you learn how to manage your time and keep the babies fed and happy, and one day you realise that the much talked about twelve weeks have gone by.

So, once the craziness subsides a little, what comes next? The twins become more alert and aware and let's face it, more fun. They will have to learn to eat, learn to sit up, and cut some teeth. They will have nappy rashes at some stage, start crawling, cry a lot, and learn to sleep through the night. It's a huge time of learning and growth.

## EARLY MILESTONES

Babies learn new things at a very fast rate and it is amazing to watch them grow and develop new skills. As with all other aspects of raising your twins, try not to compare yours too much with your friend's babies. All babies learn new skills at different rates and often hit milestones at a different time. If your twins show no signs of attempting to move about or you have any concerns at all talk to your doctor or public health team.

These are the milestones that most babies reach during their first year:

| Age | Milestones |
|-----|-----------|

**0–3 Months**  During these early months babies gradually lose that cute 'newborn' look as they become more alert-looking and start to put on weight.

By three months old your twins will have more control of their heads and wlll be able to hold them up. They will even be able to raise their heads when lying on their tummies.

**4–6 Months**  Twins make lots of discoveries at this stage: their hands, their feet, each other.

By six months old they will be able to hold things in their hands.

They will start rolling around and pushing themselves up with their arms when lying on their tummies.

**7–9 Months**  During these months babies learn to sit up on their own. They are usually all teething by now and learning how to eat solid food.

They will start crawling, sliding or shuffling along the floor.

They will be able to pick up smaller items than before and swap things from one hand to the other.

**10-12 Months**  This is an exciting stage for babies as they get much better at crawling and start pulling themselves up to standing. Some babies even get around on their feet by holding onto the furniture at this stage although most don't walk for another couple of months (our twins waited until 17 months to walk unaided).

## ECZEMA

Eczema is a skin condition which will leave your babies' skin very dry with some red itchy patches, or tiny red bumps. It's not contagious but it is itchy and uncomfortable. In babies it can usually flare up on their scalp, arms, legs or tummy. As they get older it will also appear on the backs of their knees or inside the elbows.

There are a number of factors that can cause eczema to flare up in babies (including lactose intolerance and a genetic predisposition to the condition). If you are in any way unsure about whether your twins have it or about how to treat it, or if you find the eczema doesn't clear up, then you should talk to your doctor. Chances are, they will be able to help you straight away and if they think you need it, they will refer you to a skin specialist. In the meantime and in most cases, there are some simple things you can do to manage eczema and keep your babies as comfortable as possible.

- Dress your twins in cotton. Avoid wool and 'hairy' clothes as they will irritate the skin.
- Wash clothes in detergent designed for sensitive skin.
- Avoid using bubble bath as it dehydrates the skin.
- Avoid over-bathing as soap and water also dehydrate the skin. You could always use baby lotion on cotton wool to cleanse the skin.
- Apply moisturiser after baths as the warm water opens up the pores on the skin making it easier for it to absorb moisture. Pharmacies stock some great ones that you might end up using yourself! Just watch that you are using non-perfumed, hypoallergenic, and baby friendly creams.
- You can use an emulsifying ointment (also called 'emollient cream') as soap in the bath. This can get very greasy and slippery when it gets wet so keep a tight grip on your twins, especially when lifting them out of the water.
- Dust mites can often be a trigger so keep bedrooms and play areas as clean as possible.
- Eczema can sometimes be triggered by food allergies, particularly dairy products. However, before you cut out all milk and cheese from your twins' diet and fill your cupboards with soya products and goat's milk, talk to your doctor to get proper medical advice.
- Eczema can cause the skin to feel irritated, or in some cases, itchy. You can buy small cotton mittens for the babies to

wear to prevent them from scratching themselves with their
fingernails and making their skin worse.

– Air conditioning and heating systems can dry out the air
and cause drier skin. In winter try a warmer blanket instead
of automatically turning up the heating. Do be careful
though not to overheat your babies.

– As a last resort, for severe patches, your doctor might
prescribe a mild topical steroid cream, such as 1%
hydrocortisone, for you to use in small doses. The steroid in
the cream helps reduce inflammation and redness. They do
work wonders — we called ours the 'Magic Cream'.
Sometimes moisturiser just isn't going to do it and a few
dabs of something stronger can work wonders. Use very
sparingly for no more than a few days at a time as prolonged
overuse can thin the skin.

The good news is that a lot of small children grow out of eczema
gradually until it more or less disappears in their teens. It can always
flare up again in later life in reaction to an allergy or to stress but
generally speaking, the outlook is usually good.

## GETTING HELP

It can be difficult to learn to ask for help in the beginning, especially
if you are an independent sort who likes to be able to do things for
yourself. I must admit I struggled with this. I learned very quickly
though that looking after twins is such a big job that there are times
when it just makes sense to give in and ask someone to give you a
hand. Family, friends and visitors love to feel useful so why not let
them unpack the dishwasher or load the washing machine if they
suggest it? They will be delighted that you took them up on their
offer and you will have one less thing to do.

**There are lots of other ways to get help with your twins:**

• If someone asks what they can do for you and genuinely
wants to do something that will really help you out, it can
be a great help to have meals cooked. Maybe ask if they can

bring you a frozen meal you can pop into the freezer so you
don't have to try and figure out when you are going to
squeeze in time to cook and you have one less thing to think
about.

- When visitors ask whether they can bring anything why not
ask them to pick up that litre of milk or loaf of bread on
their way over that you always seem to run out of.

- It can be very helpful to have a cleaner to help you with jobs
around the house. The fact is that with baby twins to look
after you will struggle to get any of those household chores
done while the babies are very small because they will take
up all of your time. Having someone coming to do all of the
floors and bathrooms and maybe some laundry will save
you so much time and stress. They could change the beds
and do the ironing if there is any time left over. It will be a
weight off your mind.

- There are nursing agencies that you can contact to help.
They will send out a nurse to look after the twins for a night
so that you can catch up on some much needed sleep. It can
be expensive, but you may feel that this is well worth it if
you are struggling with sleep deprivation. If you do splash
out on having a nurse come to stay then you must be strict
with yourself and stay in bed and sleep, otherwise there's no
point in paying for help.

- Lots of parents hire an au pair at this stage to help with
twins, particularly if they have other children too. You may
not want to do this as it does mean having someone else
living in your house with you, however the extra pair of
hands can be invaluable when you are trying to juggle so
much. An au pair will be able to help you with all of the
daytime feeds and may even be able to get some of that
never ending housework done, depending on your terms of
employment. If your twins have colic an au pair will be
worth their weight in gold as they can help with soothing
the babies and you don't have the stress of trying to calm
two upset newborns at once.

## NAPPY RASH

Nappy rash can flare up quickly and can be mild on some occasions and sore and uncomfortable at others and all babies are liable to end up with one at some point. The good news is that it is easy to treat and you can take simple steps to help reduce the risk of your twins developing a rash in the first place.

- Change the babies' nappies often. With twins this means you won't do much else all day but stick with it.
- Avoid using soap because it dries the skin; warm water will do just fine.
- Avoid talcum powder as it can dry out and irritate the skin.
- Pop a disposable nappy liner into the nappy — it will help keep skin drier
- A lot of books and websites also recommend leaving the babies' nappy off for a while to let some air get to the skin.
- If the rash is very bad you can buy special creams in your local pharmacy to treat it, or in severe cases you should bring the twins to see your doctor.

## TEETHING

It started for us when my twins were three months old. My mum was visiting one day and we noticed the babies were unsettled and out-of-sorts. They were cranky, crying, and I couldn't find anything wrong so to be on the safe side we pottered around to our family doctor. She checked them over and finally turned to me with an apologetic grin and said 'sorry, it looks like they're teething'. Teething! I couldn't believe it but actually in hindsight the signs were there, rosy red cheeks and both babies fussing and whimpering and gnawing on their bottles. As a first-time mum though, I had nothing to compare it to, no other experience to draw on. So how would you know, especially if they start teething as early as that. After all of that it took another two months for the first tooth to arrive.

In most cases teething starts at around five or six months and I know other mums whose babies didn't start teething until seven months or later.

## Teething Remedies

So what can you do when the teething starts? There are a few remedies that you can try out to help sooth those poor aching gums.

Cold things to chew on can help to sooth inflamed gums. You can refrigerate soothers or teething rings. Cold, clean, damp face-cloths work wonders too. You can keep spare ones in the fridge ready for when the next one is required. Just don't freeze soothers because they will be too hard and the freezing soother will burn little gums.

Chewing applies pressure to the gums which distracts babies from the pain and soreness. You can use room temperature soothers or sterilised chew-toys and teething rings. It is probably best to avoid gel-filled toys as they might become damaged by the constant chewing and start to leak.

Topical gels and creams can offer some relief from the pain, although our twins just tended to lick the gel off their gums so they were fairly ineffective.

When all else fails and the pain is really bad you can administer Calpol which contains paracetamol in a pink syrup (or some other similar product). Sometimes the pain is just too bad, especially at night. Follow the guidelines on the packaging carefully and use as a last resort. The twins will be cutting lots of teeth and experts say it's best to avoid getting into the habit of dishing out the Calpol every time if you can help it.

## The Order Teeth Come In

Baby teeth usually arrive in the following order:

- Lower front incisors
- Upper front incisors
- Upper lateral incisors

- Lower lateral incisors
- First upper molars
- First lower molars
- Upper canines
- Lower canines
- Lower second molars
- Upper second molars

## Caring for Baby Teeth

It is very important to look after the baby teeth because these teeth guide in the adult teeth. If they are damaged the bone behind the teeth can also be damaged, as we discovered on a recent trip to the dentist when one of our twins fell and hurt his two front teeth. We had to monitor his front teeth very closely for a while because our dentist was concerned that any damage caused to the bone could later harm the adult teeth. Tooth decay can also cause harm to the bone and future adult teeth. You don't need to brush your baby or toddler's teeth after every rice cake or piece of toast, but a good brush morning and evening will be fine. Young children love learning to do things for themselves so introducing toothbrushes at bedtime shouldn't pose too many problems. Avoid giving them sugary drinks or cereals and limit sweet treats to special days. A treat is only a treat if they don't have it too often. Dentists also recommend that you don't give fruit juices to babies in a bottle or baby cup.

## TELEVISION

Much has been said and written about this subject. I'm sure you've met the families who strictly do not ever watch television. You have probably also come across the families whose television is on all day from morning until night. It is worth taking a few minutes to consider the pros and cons of letting small children watch television. The more you know, the better equipped you will be to make your own decision about how much television time you will allow in your house.

There is good news and bad news. The bad news has been the subject of many studies and much research and is fairly well documented. It seems that too much television for small children can lead to social, emotional and behavioural problems later on.

- Small children develop language and social skills through playing and interacting with others. Time spent watching television leaves less time for play.
- Children also need to move around a certain amount during the day. Too much time spent sitting in front of the television can both increase the risk of obesity and get in the way of learning how to roll around, crawl and walk when they are very young.
- Too much TV can disturb sleep. Our twins have disturbed nights when they have dreamt about harmless cartoons they have seen, they would have had nightmares had they watched anything scary or violent.
- Children who are used to watching lots of television can have difficulty listening and concentrating at school.
- Another huge concern is exposure to violence as children are more likely to show aggressive behaviour later on if they were regularly exposed to violent programmes when they are small.

Thankfully there is some good news too.

- Once children are over age 2 watching television can be educational and they learn about numbers, colours, wildlife, nature and the world around them.
- Watching television can also inspire and feed the imagination as children encounter wonderful characters and stories.
- And finally, it has been my experience that a short time spent watching cartoons can restore some peace when the twins are getting tired and frazzled. There are times, usually later on in the day, when some 'time-out' watching cartoons can calm everyone down and give them some much needed down time.

So the question remains, should you let your twins watch television? It seems that a few supervised cartoons once in a while will do no harm, and may even be of benefit, while too much time spent in front of the TV will do the opposite. There are also many great educational programmes designed specifically for young children that are excellent and are designed to educate and inspire children. The trick is to monitor what your twins are watching, how long they watch it for, and what effects that the programmes have on them. Turn the television off after the programme has finished and keep television as a treat rather than the norm, and they will appreciate it a lot more. You can also chat to your twins about what they have been watching. In the end it boils down to moderation and supervision.

## TRAVELLING WITH TWINS

When our twins were four months old we braved a long weekend away with them in a baby-friendly hotel. It was the best thing we could have done. The change of scenery gave us all a lift and surviving with twins in a new environment gave my confidence a huge boost. Knowing that we could not only leave the house with the babies, take a road trip, and stay overnight somewhere else, but that we could thrive on it too, was great for our morale and felt like a huge achievement.

We went for four days and it took almost as long to pack the car but it was well worth the effort. Babies require a lot of equipment in the early days and a lot of it ends up coming with you on long journeys: travel cots, blankets, nappies and nappy changing gear, bottles, formula and sterilisers, as well as toys, teddies and spare clothes. Not forgetting two small little bags for ourselves squeezed into the last inch of space leftover in the car after everything else was crammed in.

It was fun to have a few days away from the normal routine and away from the list of jobs that always need to be done. We relaxed and spent time playing with the twins and having lovely meals served to us and no washing up to do! It is easy to fall into the trap of thinking that twins are too hard to manage away from home, that they wouldn't sleep well or feed well or that it wouldn't be a break. A change of scenery is always a break even if it is just for one day or one night. It can build you up and put everything back into perspective.

## WHEN TO GO TO THE DOCTOR

One of the things that can be difficult to decide at home on your own is when to pack the kids into the car for a trip to the doctor. Really the only guide is that if you are worried, then go. You know your twins best so you really are the one who knows when something is wrong. If you are concerned about a cough, or a rash, or sore parts, or anything at all, then go and seek medical advice. No-one minds if it turns out to be a false alarm. It's better to go and be reassured than to stay at home and find out later on that there is something wrong.

There are a few obvious things to watch out for in particular:

✓ a temperature for more than 24 hours
✓ fever which drops then rises again
✓ a rash of spots that are still visible when pressed
✓ vomiting accompanied by dizziness and headaches
✓ diarrhoea in very young babies
✓ laboured breathing
✓ sore ears

## THE FIRST BIRTHDAY

The first birthday is an enormously happy milestone with twins and it's more than just a birthday. It represents the end of a tough and challenging year and the start of an exciting, and easier, new one.

You've made it! One full year later, here you are ready to celebrate the twins' first birthday. A year ago you couldn't imagine this day, it seemed like you'd never get past the madness of the first few months. Life with twins is intense, the hustle and bustle of two babies concentrated into one year. They are definitely more than the sum of their parts, as my mum used to say. So, one very busy and intense year later, here you are. Are you planning a birthday party? We did, and if I'm honest the party was really for me. We invited our families round for champagne and chocolate cake to help us celebrate reaching this milestone in our family's life. I highly recommend it! Break out the bubbly, light those birthday candles, and celebrate reaching a huge moment and a happy day.

# 8

# All About You

## IDENTITY

It is very difficult to set aside any time for yourself during that busy first year with twins. You are so preoccupied with looking after two tiny babies day and night, all the while trying to keep up with basic household chores, keep a certain amount of laundry clean, and squeeze in a bit of time with your partner if the babies happen to sleep during the evening. Somewhere in all the craziness you can very easily lose sight of yourself and what makes you *you*. It is quite common for people to lose confidence, although they rarely admit it and you wouldn't know by looking in from the outside. It is so important to take some steps early on to avoid an identity crisis later.

## Time Out

Have you had time to sit down for a few minutes with a cup of tea today? If so, you are doing an amazing job. If not, go and put the kettle on now. It is very important to make some time for yourself during the day. You need this time. It doesn't matter how many jobs need to be done. Those jobs will still be there in ten minutes time and even if you do get those jobs done there will be as many other ones waiting for you. If you get a chance to sit down for a few minutes take it. Put your feet up, flick through a book or a paper, or take the opportunity to grab the TV remote and flick through your favourite channels even if for no other reason than to have something else to talk about. It really does help to keep your mind interested and active and it will help you feel a bit more like your old self.

Have some chocolate, make a sandwich or even close your eyes. It really doesn't matter what you do as long as you take a few minutes out for yourself. You will feel rejuvenated and happier for it and if you feel happier, then your twins will too.

## New Clothes

Yes, I know this sounds shallow, but if you are feeling a little less confident, a new pair of jeans that fit properly will do wonders for your self esteem. I found I had lots of clothes, but nothing to wear after my twins were born. Maternity clothes were stretched beyond recognition and pre-baby clothes were laughably small, tops too short to cover the leftover bump and trousers that I had no hope of fitting into. A couple of long tops and a new pair of jeans did the trick nicely.

## Hair

A good haircut can do the same thing. If you don't feel brave enough for a radical change, just book yourself in for a conditioning treatment and a trim. You will benefit from the time out, the luxury of having someone else do your hair, and the new hairdo (whether a trim or a complete restyle) will boost your confidence.

## Exercise

The many health benefits of exercise have been well-documented. Exercise helps increase oxygen supply to your blood stream, helps keep your heart healthy, and releases endorphins which make you feel good afterwards. In fact a very short trawl on the internet revealed lots of physical, emotional, psychological, and mental benefits.

**The main advantages of taking regular exercise are that it:**

✓ Helps you keep your weight down. After having twins I'm sure you will be interested in this one. Exercising burns calories and the more you exercise, the more calories you burn.
✓ Is very good for your health[15].
✓ Helps lift your spirits.

✓ Gives you an energy boost.
✓ Helps you to relax and sleep better.
✓ Is fun.
✓ Relieves stress.

There are many ways to squeeze in even small amounts of exercise. There are many short exercise programmes available on the internet and YouTube has plenty of short videos that you can follow. If you have someone to look after your twins and would rather be outside, walking and running are great ways to get up and moving. You can walk or run for whatever amount of time you have available, and don't need to spend a fortune on expensive gear to get started. Most gyms nowadays will work with you to tailor-make a training programme specifically designed for you. If running and lifting weights don't appeal to you, then cycling and swimming are also great low-impact activities with many benefits.

If you don't fancy any of that and don't have anyone to mind the twins, pop them into the pram and head out with them for a walk. It takes a bit of organisation to get half an hour free to do this, but it's worth it to get out and get some fresh air. There are many ways to get moving, you just need to figure out when you are going to have time and choose something you will enjoy. It is important to remember to look after yourself so that you can give your best care to your twins.

## SLEEP

I know how tough this one is. As someone who needs a lot of sleep, I really struggled with the lack of sleep in the beginning. Even with my husband sharing the night feeds we were still up a lot at night when the twins were very small. I remember the first night I slept for four hours in a row. I knew something was different the instant I woke up; it took a while to figure out that the difference was I actually felt like I had slept for the first time in weeks. Sleep deprivation is a form of torture and has allegedly been used by a wide range of groups ranging from the ancient Romans to the CIA to wring information from their suspects and prisoners of war. I imagine it must be fairly effective.

So if you feel like your brain has been smothered in fog and you just can't think straight go easy on yourself. You are a completely normal person feeling the effects of sleep deprivation. If you feel you just can't cope with so little sleep there are a few things you can do.

- It's such a cliché now and I know you will laugh at the suggestion, but if the babies happen to nap at the same time, put your head down and doze while they are sleeping. If you really are struggling with sleep-deprivation then you need to try and rest as much as possible whenever the opportunity arises. Housework will always be there, opportunities to rest will not.
- Call in family and friends to look after the twins for a few hours during the day while you go back to bed to sleep. You will have to be strict with yourself — no getting out of bed if you hear a baby crying. Get some good earplugs and trust your family to look after the twins while you get a couple of hours of much-needed sleep. Even if you do this once a week the extra sleep will help.
- Get your partner to take turns with doing the night feeds with you and maybe see if you can get a close friend or relative to come and stay over one night to take a turn with one of the babies so that you can catch up a little on that precious sleep.
- There are nursing agencies that you can contact to help. They will send out a nurse to look after the babies for a night so that you can sleep through. It can be expensive, but you may feel that this is well worth it to catch up. Again you must be strict with yourself and stay in bed and sleep, otherwise there's no point in paying for help.

## THE WEEPS VS. POSTNATAL DEPRESSION

One of the many things I was totally unprepared for was the effect it would all have on my hormones. I shouldn't have been so surprised really. The midwife on my antenatal course did say that the 'weeps' usually set in around day three after the baby is born. I'm not the best at coping with tiredness at the best of times and I had just had twins. So why was I so surprised when the tears arrived on day four? Some celebrities in recent times have been quite open about struggling to stop crying after their babies were born or even battling more serious cases of postnatal depression, but this is still an area most people don't talk about.

## The Weeps

Apparently, as many as up to 80% of mothers can experience baby blues after the birth of their baby[16]. The 'Blues' or 'Weeps' usually set in between days three and five and coincide with breast milk starting to come in and the hormonal changes that go with that. Mothers can feel weepy, and have a lack of confidence around the twins. It is perfectly natural and does subside after a few weeks.

You have lost your independence, you can't make a cup of tea or nip to the shops, you don't fit into any of your old clothes and you are responsible for the care of two tiny babies whose only method of communication is to cry. Really when you think about it, it's no wonder most women feel a bit weepy for the first while.

All of that can seem very remote though when you are hearing about it in ante-natal classes and you do expect to sail out of hospital with two beautiful babies that you adore and are already handling really well. Reality is quite different. There are many reasons why you are not in control of your emotions —

- Your body has been through a major shock. You have just gone from being pregnant, to being a mother of two babies and you have to readjust to being just 'you' again and not three people wrapped in one. Your internal organs have to get themselves back into place where they belong. If you have a caesarean section you will be just about up and about on your feet, never mind anything else. Usually when anyone returns home after having major surgery they wrap themselves up in cotton wool and hibernate until they are ready to venture back out. After a caesarean section to have twins you return home with two newborn babies that need to be fed and winded and changed and cuddled at any time of the day or night.

- You will need some help with looking after the babies in the early weeks and this can be hard to take when you are used to being independent. I am quite independent by nature and don't always find it easy to ask for help. I knew I needed to with the twins though and shamelessly drafted in friends and family to come to the house for a few hours every afternoon to lend a hand. Nevertheless I did really look forward to the time when I would be able to manage my twins all day on my own. Needing help makes you feel less in control and this can affect your mood.
- You will be severely sleep deprived and this of all things can make anyone a little loopy. It is so important to try and get someone to help you in the beginning when you are feeding almost as often at night as you are during the day. The good news is that this phase doesn't last and very soon you will be able to sleep much more at night than you are doing now.
- Your hormones will be in overdrive. I used to think I was quite a 'stable' person not given to emotional swings and roundabouts. So it came as an enormous shock to the system to be hit by a deluge of emotions a few days after the twins were born. I just couldn't stop crying. I couldn't have even said there was anything wrong or given any reason for the tears which made it all the more frustrating. I'm not a public crier at all and felt humiliated and frustrated and confused because this wasn't how my maternity leave was supposed to start. I had seen other mums with new babies looking relaxed and happy and in control in coffee shops and here I was confined to the house with the twins during the day in that first month with the three of us taking turns to cry. I discovered this was normal and it didn't last. It gradually lifted and I eventually began to venture out and feel more in control of things. If you feel like this, don't feel ashamed or embarrassed. It's normal and it won't last.
- You have two new people in your life who depend on you for everything. It is impossible to describe the love and protective instinct you have for them. They are so dependent and vulnerable that it's frightening. So you spend every minute of your time trying to live up to that

responsibility. Thankfully you are so busy with twins in the beginning that you gradually stop panicking about things like this and just get on with the job of looking after them.

## Postnatal Depression

So when are the weeps not the weeps but actually postnatal depression? Postnatal depression is a widely-used term and is not to be confused with the weeps. There is a big difference between having a cry at some point in the day, and the devastation of feeling like you are completely out of control and that it's never going to get better. My experience with the weeps lasted for a few weeks and even then there were days when I was so tired the water-works were turned on for barely any reason at all. But through it all I knew it wouldn't last and that I just had to bide my time, sit it out and it would all get better. I still cared about the fact that the only clothes I could fit into were maternity ones and I still wanted to have the worktops clean and shining if someone was calling to the house. Sufferers of postnatal depression typically stop caring about general appearances and housework, feel anxious and fearful, find it very difficult to cope, and sometimes select a single area to home-in on and obsess about. It can strike at any time and might take you by surprise at six months, just when you are thinking you've figured it all out.

Postnatal depression can affect one in ten women[17] and can also affect men. It can affect absolutely anyone irrespective of background. The most common signs are:

- not eating
- not sleeping
- extreme tiredness and lethargy
- blurred vision or headaches
- difficulty concentrating
- struggling to make decisions
- being negative or indifferent to your husband or partner, and your twins
- not coping in any way with the daily chores and tasks of minding babies
- obsessive fears

- inability to look forward to anything
- anxiety which can lead to panic attacks
- feeling unable to cope
- feeling guilty about feeling unable to cope
- feeling like your brains have been swapped for cotton wool
- feeling that you are not yourself

Postnatal depression can start straight away but might not develop until four to six weeks after the birth, or even four to six months. It can start suddenly with no warning and can be lonely, and devastating. It can be caused by a combination of factors such as hormones, the stress of looking after two new babies, a difficult labour or an emergency caesarean section. You are more at risk of developing postnatal depression if you have had a history of depression or have had depression during your pregnancy.

Remember this is a temporary illness that you can recover from if you get some help. If you don't get help the symptoms of postnatal depression can stay with you for months. This is not the time to be stubborn and try to stick it out on your own, you need help to get better, and your family need you to get help to get better. It is so important to talk. Talking to other people will help you feel less like you are the only one struggling. You really don't have to suffer in silence.

---

*There are many people you can talk to such as your doctor, public health nurse, family, Multiple Births Association phone support, your friends, or your partner. Start small, talk to someone you trust, and with their support get help.*

---

## GOING BACK TO WORK VS. STAYING AT HOME

Like all good things in life maternity leave doesn't last forever. The first few days and weeks seem endless and then time starts to speed up. Days roll into weeks and into months and gathers speed until suddenly you realise it's time to do the sums to see whether you need to start investigating child minding options or whether you are going to stay at home. With twins this decision seems to creep up on you with astonishing speed.

Whether or not to return to work is probably one of the biggest decisions you will make during the twins' first year. Of course the decision might be made for you, whether for financial or other reasons, in which case you will be spared hours, days and weeks of agonising over what to do and whether you've made the right choice.

Some people can't get back to work quickly enough; others want to stay at home no matter what even if it means living on beans on toast. The main thing to remember is that there is no right or wrong answer. Both options have pros and cons and it's really up to you to decide what's best for your family. Always remember that as long as you base your decision on what is best for you all, then you have absolutely no reason at all to feel guilty. You probably will feel guilty anyway as all mums seem destined to do. But you have no reason to feel guilty and don't let anyone tell you otherwise.

No-one can make this decision for you but it can definitely help to think it through from all angles first.

## Staying at home

Staying at home was always referred to as 'The Dream' by the women where I worked who had kids in crèche. I remember they would talk wistfully about 'The Dream' as they managed their workload and kept the household going and raced away each day to collect their kids. A lot of crèches seem to charge extra if mums are a few minutes late for their collection time and trying to get out of work on time for public transport that may or may not be late for unspecified reasons can cause real stress. Staying at home saves all the anxiety of being away from the kids all day and all the stress of getting to the crèche on time in the evening.

Staying at home has other benefits too. You can get all of your meals cooked and household chores done during the week and have time to spend together as a family in the evening or at the weekend. Our kids are usually in bed by half seven so my husband and I have time to relax together in the evenings. We can take our time over dinner, watch TV, or each have time for hobbies. I joined the local gym and took up running. I don't have to spend the whole weekend cleaning bathrooms and unloading the washing machine. Instead, we can have family days out, or pursue hobbies, or just kick back and relax together. Our free time is really that, free time.

The truth is staying at home can be tough too. 'The Dream' is hard work. You feed and wind babies all day, juggling housework with soothing babies. When you go out to work you can have nice coffees, meet friends for lunch and even make the occasional phone call. However, if you stay at home you will be so busy that you will often feel that you don't have time for any of that. The jobs don't stop just because the babies are asleep. There will always be laundry to do and bottles to sterilise. There are no tea breaks either, or flexi-time or sick leave.

The main issues that most mums I've spoken to who opted to stay at home have had to deal with revolve around isolation, lack of intellectual stimulation, a drop in confidence and frustration at not earning their own money anymore.

Isolation is a tricky one to deal with and one that takes a lot of people by surprise. When I was pregnant with the twins I had all sorts of expectations about what life at home would be like. I thought I would be able to relax in coffee shops, go shopping, and learn to make bread. The reality of staying at home with twins is quite different. You rarely see your old friends and have to start over again making friends with other mums at mother and toddler groups. Sometimes things go so disastrously wrong that by the time you are all finally ready to go out, it's too late to go. You can easily end up spending long periods of time alone when you are so busy looking after two babies and you might not see another adult until your husband or partner gets home from work. Friends who had their babies one at a time say that they used to watch the clock waiting for their husband or partner to come home. With twins I definitely did that in the beginning. The days can be very long, especially if you've been up since five or six in the morn-ing after three hours sleep and no company all day other than Peppa Pig and some talking trains. Twins are double the work and it took me a while to get to the stage where we could go out to the shops. I did learn to make bread but it was a while after I had given up work and the twins were about two years old. And I did get out to coffee shops, just not nearly as soon as I had thought I would.

Lack of intellectual stimulation is something many people say they also struggled with in the beginning. Making the adjustment from having a successful career, to being at home all day can be hard to do. It isn't always easy to go from holding down a job where you were busy, intellectually stimulated, maybe managed a team and ran projects, to the world of nappies and sleep deprivation. I found myself singing along to cartoons and before long knew all the words to 'Bob the Builder' — chorus and both verses. An accomplishment of sorts I guess, but not quite on the same level as using your brain at work all day.

One of the many things people don't tell you while you are pregnant is that many people say they lost a little of their confidence just after their baby was born. It's no surprise that issues around isolation and not using your brain as much when you choose to stay at home can also add to a dip in confidence if you let them. It can happen to anyone whether you are having one baby or two (or three). It's a strange thing though, because having children is the most life-affirming thing you can possibly do and having twins should be twice the affirmation. But for some reason, some people lose some of their confidence. This definitely happened to me. Whether it was the fact that I couldn't remember what day it was and didn't have enough adult company, or whether I had nothing to wear and had to go and buy bigger clothes, I don't know. But it did happen and I know I wasn't alone. I also feared that others would view my decision to stay at home as a soft option. Society does have a tendency to rate people's intelligence by their current employment. Did that mean I would be viewed as less intelligent? After struggling with this for a while I decided in the end not to worry about it. I know myself how challenging and how rewarding it can be to stay at home your twins.

Staying at home obviously means that you are no longer out there earning a salary and this can be quite a difficult adjustment to make. Becoming financially dependent is quite a challenge after years of paying your own way. It helps to be pragmatic in your approach to this old chestnut. Your contribution to the household is minding the twins all day and being there for them. You may not be earning money directly, but you are saving it by not paying child-minding fees. Add this to savings in additional dry-cleaning costs you would incur if you were working, as well as the extra petrol, takeaway lunches, transport costs, and hiring a cleaner, and you may find that your financial situation wouldn't be all that different if you were working anyway. It is easier to quantify a contribution when it arrives in the form of a paycheque, but it doesn't make an intangible contribution in the form of savings on bills any less valuable. It is also worth checking out whether there are any tax breaks available to you such as a home carer's allowance, or any joint-assessment advantages for income tax.

## Going back to Work

However, staying at home with small babies is not everyone's idea of fun either. There are days when it would definitely be easier to hand the babies over to a child-minder or nanny, head off into the office, and meet the girls for lunch. No, it's definitely not everyone's cup of tea and the early months of maternity leave are an ideal time to see whether it's yours or not.

If you enjoy your career and don't think cartoons will offer enough intellectual stimulation then you shouldn't feel guilty at all about going back to work. If you feel you would like to go back to work then you should. You will be happier and therefore your twins will be happier. Staying at home will only leave you feeling down and eventually resentful. It will sap your confidence and most importantly of all could affect your relationship with your partner and your twins.

You might also feel that you want to work to help support your family. You might have special skills and be well respected at work and don't want to give that up. There is nothing wrong with this at all and you will be helping to set an example for your children and showing them how to be disciplined and work hard. You will be working hard though. It will mean having two full-time jobs, that of a mother, and that of your career. It might help to get a cleaner to help keep the house in order and save you some time at weekends.

Staying at home is often not an option nowadays. If staying at home isn't an option for you, you won't be on your own. These days most people have to work to make ends meet. If you are going back to work because you need to remember that there are probably other women where you work who have been through this same experience and can help you through it. Most women I know who have had to go back to work say they have ended up in tears in the ladies' bathroom a few times a day during the first week back. They feel guilty and miss their baby. They realise they don't feel quite as confident as they did before they left. They feel overwhelmed physically and emotionally by the change and by having to make a big adjustment all over again. You will feel this doubly so because you have two little people that you don't want to leave behind. You are not alone. You will definitely find it easier as time goes by. And you are not a bad mother!

The first day back is the hardest. Most of the mothers where you work will have felt exactly the same way when they first came back to work. Even after a holiday lots of people forget their passwords and how to log back on to their computer when they come back. You have been out of work for an extended time and your life has changed utterly. You left the office pregnant and have now come back in as a mother of two (two!) babies. You haven't had a minute to yourself since the twins were born and probably still are not getting enough sleep. You are not the same person anymore; you have experienced a total transformation of your life as you knew it. So if you find yourself looking at your computer on your first day back with no clue how to switch it on or what to do with it when you find the on switch, then remember you are not alone.

It will take you a little while to figure out how to marry the two and manage being your 'mum' self at home and your business self at work. It's a balancing act that will continue all your life. You have so much to juggle, being a partner, being a mother, being an employee, a work colleague, a sister, a friend. You have to balance doing a day's work with spending the evening with your kids, cooking, laundry, budgeting your household expenses and trying to fit in a bit of time with your husband and friends. Nevertheless, as I keep saying, it will get easier. The more you practise anything, the better you get at it. You will adjust and find out how to fit it all in. You will get better at dropping off the twins in the morning to their childminder or Day-care and getting your work done in the office and at the same time having dinner organised in advance and the laundry done. The beginning is always hardest. It will get easier. Just remember how overwhelmed you were when you first came home from hospital with the twins. Now you are managing the twins and holding down a career.

## Things it's OK to Say

- No
- Help
- Why didn't they come with instructions!
- I need chocolate
- I need to sleep
- Will they ever stop crying? *(Yes, they will!)*
- I haven't a clue what I'm doing *(Most people feel like this in the beginning! You are not alone and you will figure it out)*
- Will it ever get any easier? *(Yes it will!)*

*While I have been off work I have met lots of amazing women who go about their daily routines and don't think they are particularly special or inspiring. But they have done inspiring things like run marathons, or run the local mother and toddler group. None of these women think they are particularly amazing but I for one couldn't run a marathon. They all said they just fell into doing all of these things whether by just going for a short run at the weekend, or taking an interest in events in their community.*

*Having said that, friends who subsequently had a singleton baby said they couldn't imagine how I managed with twins. Someone thinks you are amazing to manage twins. Remember this the next time you feel a little overwhelmed or under confident and are looking at other people wondering how they manage to do those amazing things. Someone is looking at you and wondering how you do it. You are inspiring.*

# APPENDIX 1

# Exercises

During pregnancy the abdominal muscles lose strength and the muscles across your tummy spread to make room for your expanding womb. If you have a caesarean section then your core will be incredibly weak afterwards. You can do some gentle exercises to help build these muscles back up and strengthen your core again. Don't forget to talk to your doctor before starting any exercises, and wait until six weeks after your surgery before returning to any form of more strenuous exercise. Remember you have had major surgery which needs time to heal properly.

## Early Core Exercise

I went to see a Physiotherapist about my knee last year and she told me I should have been doing this core exercise after I had my twins. It seems that strengthening your core will help support your whole body, from protecting your lower back to supporting you while you walk.

Lie on your back or your side with your knees bent, whichever is more comfortable. Take a breath in, and as you breathe out slowly and gently draw in your tummy. Hold for 5 seconds and gently release. Remember to keep breathing as you count.

You can try holding the count for a few seconds longer when you get better at doing this exercise.

## Pelvic Floor Exercise

This exercise can be performed anywhere and in any position. Imagine that you need to stop yourself from going to the toilet and squeeze without squeezing your legs or bum. Hold the lift for as long as you can and release. Rest and repeat. Don't forget to breathe normally during the exercise.

## Walking

Walking will be a challenge for the first few days as you no longer have the abdominal strength you need to support your back and legs. Don't give up and try to walk around when you can.

## Circulation

This simple ankle stretch is great for your circulation and it also helps reduce any swelling. Sit with your legs stretched out in front of you making sure your back is supported. Circle your ankle for 20 seconds, concentrating on one leg at a time.

## Breathing Exercises

These are great to help with circulation and are especially important if you have had an anaesthetic.

Take a deep breath in through your nose, hold for two or three seconds, and slowly release the breath through your mouth.

# APPENDIX 2

# Recipes for Hungry Babies

Once you have successfully introduced your twins to a range of fruits and vegetables it can be helpful to have a few versatile recipes up your sleeve. The following five recipes can each be made or combined with other ingredients in three different ways giving you a total of fifteen options altogether. They can be adapted to suit individual likes and dislikes, and whatever you have in your fridge that day. If you don't have or like one of the ingredients simply leave it out, or put something else in instead. They can be made fresh each time, or cooked in big batches and frozen in little portions ready to defrost when you need them.

## 1 – Steamed Root Vegetable Puree

*Once you have introduced root vegetables, start combining them to create different flavour combinations. The mixture can be pureed for babies who can't chew, and left lumpier as the twins get bigger and start to be able to chew their food. You can double or treble these quantities to make extra which can be frozen for future meals.*

*They also make a great side dish for the grown-ups.*

*Choose any two or three root vegetables:*

- 1 × sweet potato
- ¼ × butternut squash
- 1 × medium sized parsnip
- ½ × small turnip
- 1 × medium sized carrot

*Method*

- Peel the selected vegetables and chop into small pieces.
- Steam your chosen vegetables for fifteen minutes or until soft.
- Puree with a little cooled boiled water.

## Option 1

Select any combination of vegetables and cook as described. Sweet potato and parsnip work well together and either turnip, parsnip and carrot, or butternut squash and carrot are more great combinations. You can mash these with a fork to create more texture and serve as a side dish for the grown-ups.

## Option 2

Cook any combination of vegetables and mash with a fork to create more texture. You can use this as a topping for any pie, for example, chicken pie (see Chicken and Broccoli recipe below for the sauce).

## Option 3

Once your twins have got the hang of eating you can cube the cooked vegetables instead of pureeing them. Serve mixed with wholegrain rice either as a side dish or on its own for a filling lunch.

# 2 – Chicken and Broccoli Puree

*This is such an adaptable recipe. You can double or treble the quantities and freeze the extra portions. You can even make a large pot of it and leave some aside before you puree it for your own meals so that you are starting to cook one meal for everyone. If you don't have any broccoli you can use peas instead.*

*When the twins are over a year old you can add a topping of breadcrumbs or pastry to make a delicious bake for all the family. At this stage you can also make an easier sauce with one small tub of crème fraiche combined with 300ml chicken stock, instead of making a white sauce. I came across this idea when making James Martin's 'Chicken and Leek Pie' recipe and find it works very well with broccoli.*

- 1 × small onion, chopped
- 25g butter
- 25g flour
- 300ml milk
- 1 × small chicken breast, skinned and boned, chopped into small pieces
- 1 × handful cooked broccoli florets
- 25g grated cheese (optional)

## Method

- Gently fry the chopped onion in a small amount of olive oil in a saucepan until translucent.
- Add the chopped chicken pieces and cook gently with the lid on until the chicken is cooked through.
- Meanwhile, in a separate pan, melt the butter over a low heat. Add the flour and combine. Add the milk slowly whisking all the time. Bring to the boil slowly and continue whisking to avoid lumps. Once the sauce has thickened remove from the heat.
- Combine the sauce, chicken and onion mixture, and broccoli. Cook for a few minutes to combine and transfer to a dish to cool. Add in the grated cheese if liked for more flavour. Puree to a smooth texture for young babies, or leave lumpy for toddlers.

## Option 1

Puree the chicken and broccoli as described above.

## Option 2

Triple the quantities and cook the chicken and broccoli mixture as described. Transfer to an ovenproof dish. Top with some grated cheese and breadcrumbs and bake for fifteen minutes or until the breadcrumbs are golden.

*Option 3*

Triple the quantities and cook the chicken and broccoli mixture as described. Add in some frozen peas (add in your own quantity according to taste). Transfer the mixture to an ovenproof dish. Sprinkle over some grated cheese and then top with either short crust or puff pastry. (You can buy these frozen at the supermarket. Simply defrost and roll out to the size of your baking dish). Bake for twenty minutes or until the pastry is golden brown.

Now that my twins are older I add raw broccoli to the sauce to make these pies and bakes. I find that cooked broccoli can sometimes go a little too soft in the oven, but raw broccoli cooks just the right amount in the pie. Either way it's just a matter of taste, you can add raw or cooked broccoli to your sauce before you bake it depending on how much you like it cooked.

## 3 – Pasta Sauce with Vegetables

*This sauce is a pureed version of one I have been making for many years and is a brilliant way to get your babies to eat vegetables without them realising it. Serve with pasta and grated cheese. Once your twins are over a year old you can add in some bacon and a teaspoon of balsamic vinegar.*

*I use these vegetables because I like them but you can add in more or different vegetables if you prefer, or substitute one if you don't have it in the fridge that day. You can also use different herbs and increase or decrease according to taste. Annabel Karmel has a different version of this recipe in her wonderful book '**New Complete Baby and Toddler Meal Planner**' (Ebury Press, 2007)', and there are dozens of alternative versions to this recipe online. They all use different ingredients so if you don't have the ones listed below in your fridge, look up the other recipes for more inspiration and alternative vegetables to use.*

- Pasta
- 1 × small onion
- 1 × half clove garlic
- 75g mushrooms
- ½ a red or yellow pepper
- ⅓ courgette
- 1 × 400g tin of chopped tomatoes
- ½ × level teaspoon chopped thyme or mixed herbs

*Method*

- Cook the pasta according the instructions on the packet. Cooking methods will vary according to the type of pasta you use.
- Wash and finely chop all of the vegetables.
- Gently cook the chopped onion in a pan for five minutes or until translucent. Add the garlic and cook for one minute.
- Pour in the chopped tomatoes and the chopped vegetables.
- Cook gently for fifteen minutes or until all of the vegetables are soft.
- Once the sauce is cooked allow to cool for a few minutes. Puree to a smooth consistency adding some boiled water if the sauce is too thick, and combine with the cooked pasta.

*Option 1*

Cook as described and serve with pasta.

*Option 2*

Cook and puree the sauce as described. Spread a dessert spoon of the sauce on some wholemeal pitta bread and top with grated cheese for a quick and healthy alternative to pizza.

*Option 3*

When the twins are able to chew food you can cook the sauce and leave the vegetables a lumpier texture. Cover with a topping of the sweet potato and parsnip puree or mash (see Steamed Root Vegetable Puree) to make a comforting, filling and tasty vegetable pie.

## 4 – Vegetable Soup and Toasty Soldiers

*As soon as the babies can chew their way through toast, this is a great way to encourage them to experiment with feeding themselves. The 'soldiers' should be dipped into the soup which ensures that even the fussiest of eaters will be getting at least a few spoons-worth of vegetables, and all in the name of fun. You can vary the root vegetables used, or leave out the parsnips or potatoes if you don't have them. The soup is tasty enough for adults too so you can make it for all of the family. Once the twins are over a year old you can use vegetable or chicken stock instead of water.*

*A few years ago my friend told me she was adding ginger and a potato to her homemade soup. I tried it and have been adding them to my carrot soup ever since.*

*The soup will keep for twenty-four hours in the fridge and can be frozen in batches for another day.*

- 1 onion, chopped
- ½ inch sized piece of ginger, peeled
- 6 medium carrots
- 1 medium parsnip
- 1 medium potato or 1 medium sweet potato

## Method

- Peel and finely chop all of the vegetables.
- Gently fry the onion in a little oil for a few minutes until translucent.
- Remove the pan from the heat and grate over the ginger. Return to the heat and stir for half a minute.
- Next add the chopped vegetables and cover these with cold water. Bring the water to the boil and then turn down to a gentle simmer.
- Cook for twenty minutes or until the vegetables are soft.
- Remove from the heat and blend to a soft soup consistency adding more boiled water if necessary.
- While the soup is cooling prepare the toasty soldiers. Toast one slice of wholemeal bread and slice lengthways into thin slices.

## Option 1

Cook as described above using a normal potato and serve with toasty soldiers. For the adults you can add some black pepper and some parmesan cheese for extra flavour.

*Option 2*

Leave out the potato and onion and replace with sweet potato and a leek for a different, sweeter flavour. For the adults you can swirl in a spoonful of cream for a smooth texture and top with croutons.

*Option 3*

When the soup is cooked, add in some cooked egg noodles or pasta shapes for a filling meal.

## 5 – Roast Butternut Squash and Carrot Soup

*This soup is also great with Toasty Soldiers to encourage hungry babies and young toddlers to feed themselves and eat lots of vegetables at the same time. The soup is tasty enough for adults too so you can make it for all of the family. If you don't have time to roast the butternut squash don't worry, you can skip this step and the soup will still taste great. Simply peel and chop the butternut squash and add it with the carrots. Again, once the twins are over a year old you can use vegetable or chicken stock instead of water.*

*The soup will keep for twenty-four hours in the fridge and can be frozen in batches for another day.*

- 1 onion, chopped
- 3 medium carrots, peeled and chopped
- 1 small Butternut Squash
- 1 small potato (optional)

*Method*

- Slice the butternut squash in half lengthways, cut out the seeds, and roast in a medium oven for twenty minutes. (This will soften the squash and make it much easier to peel.)
- Gently fry the onion in a little olive oil until translucent and add in the chopped carrots, and potato (if using). Remove the butternut squash from the oven, scoop the soft flesh out of the skins and add to the onion and vegetables.
- Cover with water and simmer gently for twenty minutes, or until the carrots are soft. Remove from the heat and blend, adding more boiled water if necessary.

### Option 1

Cook as described and serve with toasty soldiers.

### Option 2

Add a teaspoon of ground cumin to the soup and serve with pitta bread and hummus.

### Option 3

Cook as described and serve as a fun and tasty dip with sliced carrots, celery and cucumber.

# APPENDIX 3

# Vaccination Programmes

## VACCINATIONS FOR BABIES

Your local health authority will run a programme of vaccinations for your babies and they are usually administered through your doctor. Most babies cry when they receive their injections so it definitely helps to have someone there with you to look after one of the twins while you hold the one who is receiving their vaccinations. Babies start their vaccinations at a few months old so that they can get the earliest possible protection from the various diseases. If your twins miss one of their vaccinations for some reason don't worry, they can catch up later although it is best to try and get them on time as much as you can. Remember, if you don't get the vaccines your twins will be at risk of contracting the diseases, and will also be at risk of passing those diseases onto others.

There are a lot of scare stories out there and you might be nervous that the vaccines will have some other terrible side effects. Studies have shown that there is no link between vaccines and autism or multiple sclerosis, or other conditions such as allergies, asthma, or attention deficit disorder[18]. These vaccinations are only given because they are safe. As ever, if you have any concerns or worries at all about any of the vaccinations, talk to your doctor or local public health nurse for more information and reassurance.

## VACCINATION PROGRAMMES

*These vaccines are listed here for information purposes only and include from birth to eighteen months old to give you an idea of what to expect during those early moths. All vaccination programmes continue on through-out childhood to give maximum protection against these serious diseases. Vaccinations schedules vary between territories and from state to state.* **Always check with your own doctor to get the most recent schedule of vaccinations for your twins.**

Vaccination programmes cover a variety of serious diseases. These are the most common vaccines and diseases covered in the various programmes during the babies' first eighteen months:

- **BCG** is a vaccination against Tuberculosis. In Ireland one vaccination injection is given to babies at birth.
- **Diphtheria** is a serious disease that can damage the heart and nervous system and can lead to severe breathing problems[19]. The vaccine for Diphtheria is often given in three doses. It is sometimes combined with other vaccines in one injection.
- **Haemophilus Influenza type b (Hib)** is bacteria which can cause diseases such as meningitis[20]. This vaccine is often administered in four doses. It can be given on its own, or sometimes combined with other vaccines in one injection.
- **Meningitis C** can cause serious damage to the brain. The Meningitis C vaccine protects against diseases caused by the group C virus.[21] The vaccine for Meningococcus C vaccination programme varies from country to country. Some states administer one injection at around 12 months and others give two or three injections.
- The **MMR** vaccine protects against Measles, Mumps and Rubella. This is usually given at around twelve months old.
- **Pneumococcal** infections can lead to lung infections, septicaemia and meningitis[22]. This vaccine is usually administered in three doses.
- **Polio** is a virus which can cause paralysis and difficulty breathing[23]. The vaccine for Polio is often given in three doses. It is sometimes combined with other vaccines in one injection.

- **Rotavirus** infections lead to diarrhoea and vomiting which in turn can lead to dehydration[24]. The vaccine is often given in two or three doses and can be given in the form of drops straight into the baby's mouth.
- **Tetanus** (also referred to as 'lockjaw') a potentially fatal disease which affects muscles and can cause severe breathing and swallowing problems[25]. This vaccine is often given in three doses and combined with other vaccines in one injection.
- **Varicella** is also called chicken pox and is included in vaccination programmes in some countries. It is usually given at age twelve to eighteen months.
- **Whooping cough**[26] causes spells of severe coughing making it difficult to breathe. It is also known as Pertussis. The vaccine is commonly given in three or four doses and is often combined with other vaccines in one injection.

# REFERENCES

## Chapter 1

1  http://scienceline.ucsb.edu/getkey.php?key=244 (accessed April 15, 2015)
2  http://www.webmd.com/baby/news/20060222/older-women-more-likely-to-have-twins (accessed May 2, 2015)
3  http://uwtwinregistry.org/do-identical-twins-always-have-the-same-hand-preference/ (accessed April 15, 2015)
4  http://www.indexmundi.com/g/r.aspx?v=25 (accessed April 15, 2015)
5  http://www.ncbi.nlm.nih.gov/pubmed/3434134 (accessed April 15, 2015)
6  http://www.acog.org/~/media/For%20Patients/faq092.pdf?dmc=1&ts=20140514T1520249990 (accessed April 15, 2015)
7  http://www.nhs.uk/conditions/pregnancy-and-baby/pages/what-causes-twins.aspx#close (accessed April 15, 2015)
8  http://www.ncbi.nlm.nih.gov/pmc/articles/PMC2840794/ (Accessed April 15, 2015)

*See also:*

http://multiples.about.com/od/funfacts/tp/howtohavetwins.htm (accessed May 5, 2015)

## Chapter 2

### Pregnant with Twins
http://www.twin-pregnancy-and-beyond.com/twin-pregnancy-week-by-week.html (accessed April 30, 2015)
http://www.coombe.ie/?nodeId=125#ultra4 (accessed April 30, 2015)

Practical Parenting 'Your Pregnancy Week by Week', foreword by Dame Karlene
    Davis, Royal College of Midwives, (Hamlyn, 2005)

## Chapter 3

9  http://www.mayoclinic.org/tests-procedures/c-section/basics/what-
    you-can-expect/prc-20014571 (accessed May 2, 2015)

### See also:

**Pain Relief**
http://www.nhs.uk/conditions/pregnancy-and-baby/pages/pain-relief-
    labour.aspx (accessed Feb 2015)
http://www.nmh.ie/labour-delivery/pain-relief-in-labour.234.html
    (accessed Feb 2015)
http://www.babycentre.co.uk/c25004189/pain-relief-in-labour (accessed
    April 15,2015)
**Natural labour**
http://www.nmh.ie/_fileupload/Community%20Midwives/CM_Labour
    %20and%20Birth%20Information_Final.pdf (accessed April 23, 2015)
www.babycentre.co.uk/a3585/giving-birth-to-twins (accessed Feb 2015)
http://www.whattoexpect.com/pregnancy/twins-and-multiples/giving-
    birth/multiple-birth-experience.aspx (accessed April 20, 2015)
**Wound Care**
National Maternity Hospital (of Ireland) 'Wound Care; patient Information
    Leaflet after Discharge'

## Chapter 4

10  http://www.mayoclinic.org/diseases-conditions/colic/basics/
    definition/con-20019091 (Accessed April 14, 2015)

### See also:

**Reusable nappies**
http://www.babycentre.co.uk/baby/buyingforbaby/nappies/reusable/
    (accessed Feb 2015)
**Bathing**
Dr Miriam Stoppard 'New Baby Care' (Dorling Kindersley, UK, 2009), pages
    70-85
**Crying**
Dr Miriam Stoppard 'New Baby Care' (Dorling Kindersley, UK, 2009), pages
    158-166

**Lactose intolerance**
http://www.ehow.com/about_5073063_signs-lactose-intolerance
babies.html (accessed April 21, 2015)
http://www.mayoclinic.org/diseases-conditions/lactose-
intolerance/basics/symptoms/con-20027906 (accessed April 17, 2015)

## Chapter 5

11  Dr Miriam Stoppard 'New Baby Care', (Dorling Kindersley, UK, 2009), p.89
12  Dr Miriam Stoppard 'New Baby Care', (Dorling Kindersley, UK, 20090, p.89
13  http://motherhood.modernmom.com/demand-vs-scheduled-breastfeeding-6278.html and
https://www2.aap.org/breastfeeding/files/pdf/tenstepsposter.pdf (accessed May 2, 2015)
14  http://www.bbcgoodfood.com/howto/guide/top-tips-freezing-food (Accessed April 14, 2015)

### See also:

**When to feed**
http://www.webmd.com/parenting/baby/features/your-babys-feeding-on-demand-or-on-schedule (accessed Feb 2015)
**Bottle feeding**
Dr Miriam Stoppard 'New Baby Care' (Dorling Kindersley, UK, 2009)
**Breastfeeding**
Dr Miriam Stoppard 'New Baby Care' (Dorling Kindersley, UK, 2009)
Emma O'Mahony 'Double Trouble, Twins and How to Survive Them' (Thorsons, 2003)
**Freezing Food**
http://www.bbcgoodfood.com/howto/guide/top-tips-freezing-food (Accessed April 14, 2015)

## Chapter 6

http://www.babycenter.com/0_parent-led-baby-schedules-baby-wise-gina-ford-and-others_3658361.bc (accessed April 15, 2015)
http://www.babycenter.com/0_baby-led-baby-schedules-sears-spock-and-others_3658355.bc (accessed April 15, 2015)
http://www.babycenter.com/0_combination-baby-schedules-supernanny-baby-whisperer-and-oth_3658358.bc (accessed May 2, 2015)

Tracy Hogg 'Secrets of the Baby Whisperer: How to Calm, Connect and Communicate with your Baby' (Ballantine Books, 2005)

## Chapter 7

**Early Milestones**
Dr Miriam Stoppard 'New Baby Care' (Dorling Kindersley, 2009), Chapter 11
http://www.mayoclinic.org/healthy-lifestyle/infant-and-toddler health/in-epth/HLV20049400 articles on infant development (accessed April 14, 2015)
**Eczema**
http://www.babycentre.co.uk/a541297/baby-eczema-causes-symptoms-treatments-and-creams (accessed Feb 2015)
http://www.patient.co.uk/health/atopic-eczema (accessed April 20, 2015)
**Nappy rash**
http://www.netdoctor.co.uk/diseases/facts/nappyrash.htm (accessed Feb 2015)
Dr Miriam Stoppard 'New Baby Care' (Dorling Kindersley, 2009), pages 68-69
http://www.patient.co.uk/health/nappy-rash (accessed May 2, 2015)
http://www.webmd.boots.com/children/baby/guide/nappy-rash-irritation (accessed May 2, 2015)
**Teething**
http://www.webmd.com/children/primary-baby-teeth-eruption-sequence (accessed April 20, 2015)
**TV**
http://www.raisesmartkid.com/all-ages/1-articles/13-the-good-and-bad-effects-of-tv-on-your-kid (accessed May 2, 2015)
http://kidshealth.org/parent/positive/family/tv_affects_child.html (accessed Feb 2015)
http://www.mayoclinic.org/healthy-living/childrens-health/in-depth/children-and-tv/art-20047952?pg=2 (accessed April 20, 2015)
http://www.med.umich.edu/yourchild/topics/tv.htm (accessed Feb 2015)

## Chapter 8

15  http://www.mayoclinic.org/healthy-living/fitness/in-depth/exercise/art-20048389?pg=1 (accessed May 2, 2015)
16  http://www.mentalhealthamerica.net/conditions/postpartum-disorders, and http://www.healthychildren.org/English/ages-stages/prenatal/delivery-beyond/Pages/Understanding-Motherhood-and-Mood-Baby-Blues-and-Beyond.aspx (accessed April , 2015)

17   http://www.hse.ie/eng/health/az/P/Postnatal-
     depression/Symptoms-of-postnatal-depression.html (Accessed April
     14, 2015)

## See also:

**Exercise**
http://www.mayoclinic.org/healthy-living/fitness/in-depth/exercise/art-
20048389?pg=1 (accessed May 2, 2015)
**Postnatal depression**
http://www.postnataldepression.com/more-information (accessed April
2015)
http://www.nhs.uk/conditions/Postnataldepression/Pages/Introduction.
aspx (accessed Feb 20150
http://www.hse.ie/eng/services/Publications/Mentalhealth/Chasing_th
e_blues_away.pdf (accessed May 2, 2015)

## Appendix 1

'*After a Caesarean Birth*' Association of Chartered Physiotherapists in
   Obstetrics and Gynaecology (leaflet)

## Appendix 2

'Chicken and Leek Pie' recipe page 87 *from* James Martin '*The Collection*',
   Mitchell Beazley, 2008

## Appendix 3

18   http://www.hse.ie/eng/health/immunisation/pubinfo/
     babychildimm/parentsguide.pdf (accessed April 30, 2015)
19   http://www.mayoclinic.org/diseases-
     conditions/diphtheria/basics/complications/con-20022303 (accessed
     April 15, 2015)
20   http://www.cdc.gov/vaccines/hcp/vis/vis-statements/hib.html
     (accessed April 15, 2015)
21   http://www.nhs.uk/Conditions/vaccinations/Pages/men-c-
     vaccine.aspx (accessed April 15, 2015)
22   http://www.nhs.uk/Conditions/vaccinations/Pages/pneumococcal-
     vaccination.aspx (accessed April 15, 2015)
23   http://www.cdc.gov/vaccines/hcp/vis/vis-statements/ipv.html
     (accessed April 15, 2015)

24  http://www.nhs.uk/Conditions/vaccinations/Pages/rotavirus-vaccine.aspx (accessed April 15, 2015)

25  http://www.cdc.gov/tetanus/about/symptoms-complications.html (accessed April 15, 2015)

26  http://www.mayoclinic.org/diseases-conditions/whooping cough/basics/symptoms/con-20023295 (accessed April 15, 2015)

*See also:*

http://www.who.int/immunization/policy/immunization_tables/en/ (accessed May 7, 2015)

http://vaccine-schedule.ecdc.europa.eu/Pages/Scheduler.aspx (accessed May 5, 2015)

## For your Bookshelf

It can be useful to have some good medical guides at home that will give you expert medical advice on how to look after your twins. I loved **Dr Miriam Stoppard's book 'New Baby Care'** (Dorling Kindersley, 2009) which offers practical advice from the first day at home up to age three. It also includes expert guidance on social and physical development at every stage.

**'Your Pregnancy Week by Week' Practical Parenting** (Hamlyn, 2005) is packed with fascinating details of the babies' development during your pregnancy. It focuses largely on singleton babies but twins follow the same development up until the end. It also has great information for mums on labour, what you might be experiencing and what to do about some of the uncomfortable symptoms you will be having.

I couldn't have managed without **Annabel Karmel's 'New Complete Baby and Toddler Meal Planner'** (Ebury Press, 2007). Annabel Karmel is the undisputed guru of baby and toddler food and her books are full of nutrition advice and great recipes for every stage. She includes meal planners for babies and toddlers which help you to ensure your twins are getting enough variety of food and avoid falling into the trap of cooking the same meals over and over again.

I was given a copy of **Emma O'Mahony's 'Double Trouble, Twins and How to Survive Them'** (Thorsons, 2003) which offers a light-hearted look at life with twins. It includes personal stories from other mums and made me giggle when I needed it.